DUSTY RICHMOND

DRUG GUIDE
for Paramedics

D0144176

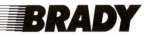

DRUG GUIDE
for Paramedics

SECOND EDITION

Richard A. Cherry, MS, NREMT-P
Clinical Assistant Professor
of Emergency Medicine
Technical Director for Medical Simulation
Upstate Medical University
Syracuse, New York

Bryan E. Bledsoe, DO, FACEP, EMT-P
Adjunct Associate Professor of Emergency Medicine
The George Washington University Medical Center
Washington, DC
and
Emergency Physician
Midlothian, Texas

Upper Saddle River, New Jersey 07458

Library of Congress Cataloging-in-Publication Data

Cherry, Richard A.
  Drug guide for paramedics / Richard A. Cherry, Bryan E. Bledsoe.—
2nd ed.
    p. cm.
  Includes index.
  ISBN 0-13-193645-X (pbk.)
    1. Drugs—Handbooks, manuals, etc. 2. Emergency medicine—
Handbooks, manuals, etc. 3. Medical emergencies—
Chemotherapy—Handbooks, manuals, etc. I. Bledsoe, Bryan E.
II. Title.
  [DNLM: 1. Pharmaceutical Preparations—administration &
dosage—Handbooks. 2. Drug Therapy—Handbooks.
3. Emergencies—Handbooks. 4. Emergency Medical Technicians—
Handbooks. QV 39 C522d 2006]
RM301.12.C45 2006
615'.1—dc22

                                                    2006043402

10 9 8 7 6
ISBN 0-13-193645-X

CONTENTS

Commonly Prescribed Medications

Brady's *Drug Guide for Paramedics* was designed with two purposes in mind. First, it serves as a convenient field guide for emergency providers of all levels by providing current, reliable information about emergency drugs and their patients' medications. Second, it serves as a supplement to the *Paramedic Care: Principles & Practice* series by providing paramedic students with comprehensive profiles of more than 100 drugs used in the emergency setting. Adapted from the top-selling *Prentice Hall Health Professional's Drug Guide 2005–2006* by Shannon, Wilson, and Stang, the guide is divided into two sections.

Section 1—Drug Profiles
The drugs in this section are alphabetized by their generic names. Each drug is profiled with the following information:

Class: This describes the class in which the drug is classified.

Trade Names: These are the trade names given to the drugs by their respective manufacturers. Canadian and Australian drugs are included.

Therapeutic Action/Pharmacodynamics: This describes the mechanism by which the specific drug produces physiologic and biochemical changes at the cell, tissue, or organ level. It also describes the expected benefits of administering this drug to the patient.

Emergency Uses/Doses: These are the indications for using the drug in the emergency setting, along with the adult and pediatric doses.

Pharmacokinetics: This section lists information about onset, peak, and duration of drug action. It also lists the mechanisms of metabolism and elimination when known.

Contraindications and Precautions: Many drugs are contraindicated and therefore should not be used in specific conditions. In other cases the drug should be used with great caution because of a greater-than-average risk of adverse effects.

Adverse/Side Effects: Virtually all drugs have adverse or side effects that may be bothersome to some individuals but not to others. In this entry, adverse/side effects are listed according to systems or organs.

Interactions: Individual drugs, drug classes, and foods that interact with the drug under discussion are listed. Drugs may interact to inhibit or enhance one another; thus drug interactions may improve the therapeutic response, lead to therapeutic failure, or produce specific adverse reactions.

Prehospital Considerations: Here, specific information regarding the prehospital use of the drug is discussed.

Section 2—Commonly Prescribed Medications

In this section, the drug classes are defined. You should become familiar with each class in order to predict for which medical condition the drug is usually prescribed. Once you know the classes, and your patient presents you with an unknown drug, simply reference it in this section of the guide. For example, knowing what a bronchodilator does and the illnesses for which it is prescribed can help you determine your patient's primary problem and make your field diagnosis.

No one can remember all the characteristics of all drugs prescribed for patients to take at home. In fact, with the approval of new drugs on a daily basis, it is impossible even to remember their names and for what ailment they are prescribed. For this reason, this section also includes an alphabetical list of hundreds of common home medications by trade and generic names. When presented with an unknown medication, you can quickly reference the drug in this section.

For quick reference, the index at the back of this pocket guide lists drugs by trade and generic names.

Brady's *Drug Guide for Paramedics* can be used by field providers before the call—to refresh their memories on emergency drug profiles and drug classes; during the call—to quickly identify their patients' home medications; and after the call—as an adjunct to accurate documentation. We hope you find this guide helpful. If you have any suggestions for the next edition, please let us know. Good luck!

Acknowledgments

Our thanks to Margaret T. Shannon, Billie Ann Wilson, and Carolyn L. Stang for their cooperation and assistance in preparation of Brady's *Drug Guide for Paramedics*. Their *Health Professional's Drug Guide* provided the foundation upon which this pocket reference is based.

Our thanks also to the following instructors for their review of manuscript. Their suggestions were helpful in preparation of this edition.

Attila Hertelendy, MS(c), MHSM, NREMT-P, CCEMT-P
University of Mississippi Medical Center
Department of Health Sciences
Jackson, MS

Scott Jones, MBA, EMT-P
Director of the Paramedic Academy
Victor Valley College
Victorville, CA

Darren Lacroix
Del Mar College,
Corpus Christi, TX

Luke Littrell, BA, NREMT-P
Eastern Iowa Community College District
Davenport, IA

Bill Locke
EMS Instructor/Coordinator
Moraine Park Technical College
Fond du Lac, WI

Michael W. Lynch, NREMT-P, CCEMT-P
Administrative Director
Crozer Chester Medical Center
EMS Training Institute
Upland, PA

Brittany Martinelli, BSRT-NPS, NREMT-P
Santa Fe Community College
Gainesville, FL

Mike McLaughlin
Director of Health Education
Kirkwood Community College
Cedar Rapids, IA

John Rinard
EMS Program Supervisor
Texas Engineering Extension Service
College Station, TX

Richard A. Cherry
Bryan E. Bledsoe

Drug Profiles

ABCIXIMAB

Classes: IIb–IIIa glycoprotein inhibitor; antithrombotic; antiplatelet

Trade Name: ReoPro

Therapeutic Action/Pharmacodynamics: Abciximab binds to the IIb–IIIa glycoprotein receptors found on platelets and vessel wall endothelial and smooth muscle cells. This inhibits platelet aggregation by preventing fibrinogen and other adhesive molecules from binding with receptors on activated platelets.

Emergency Use: Abciximab is used, in addition to aspirin, as an adjunct to percutaneous coronary intervention to prevent cardiac ischemic complications. *Adult dose:* Unstable angina (prior to PTCA): 250 mcg/kg IV followed by maintenance dose of 10 mcg/min for 18–24 hr. *Pediatric dose:* Determined on case-by-case basis (rarely used).

Pharmacokinetics

Absorption: Immediate with IV administration; >90% inhibition of platelet aggregation within 2 hr; duration is 48 hr; half-life is 30 min.

Distribution: Well distributed in all body fluids.

Contraindications and Precautions: Because abciximab may increase the risk of bleeding, it is contraindicated in the following clinical situations: active internal bleeding; recent (within 6 weeks) GI or GU bleeding of clinical significance; history of stroke within 2 yr or stroke with a significant residual neurological deficit; thrombocytopenia; recent (within 6 weeks) major surgery or trauma; intracranial neoplasm, arteriovenous malformation, or aneurysm; severe uncontrolled hypertension; presumed or documented history of vasculitis.

Adverse/Side Effects: Heme: Bleeding, including intracranial, retroperitoneal, and hematemesis; thrombocytopenia. • CNS: Dizziness, anxiety, abnormal thinking, agitation, hypesthesia, confusion, muscle contractions, coma, hypertonia, diplopia. • Respiratory: Pneumonia, rales, pleural effusion, bronchitis, bronchospasm, pleurisy, pulmonary embolism, rhonchi. • M/S: Myalgia. • GU: Urinary retention, dysuria, abnormal renal function, frequent micturition, cystalgia, urinary incontinence, prostatitis.

Interactions: Oral anticoagulants, NSAIDS, dipyridamole, ticlopidine, dextran may increase risk of bleeding.

Prehospital Considerations

- Monitor for signs and symptoms of bleeding at all potential sites (e.g., catheter insertion, needle puncture; GI, GU, or retroperitoneal sites); hypersensitivity that may occur any time during administration.
- Avoid or minimize unnecessary invasive procedures and devices to reduce risk of bleeding.
- If symptoms of an allergic reaction or anaphylaxis appear, stop the infusion immediately and give the appropriate treatment.
- Although no incompatibilities have been shown with IV infusion fluids or commonly used cardiovascular drugs, administer abciximab in a separate IV line whenever possible and not mixed with other medications.

Acetaminophen

ACETAMINOPHEN

Classes: Analgesic; antipyretic

Trade Names: Abenal (Can), Acephen, Aceta, Actamen, Actimol (Can), Anacin-3, Anuphen, Apacet, APAP, Atasol (Can), Banesin, Dapa, Datril, Dolanex, Dorcol, Dymadon (Aus), Exdol (Aus), Feverall, Genapap (Can), Genebs, Halenol, Liquiprim, Mapap, Medacap, Neopap, Oraphen, Panadol, Panamax (Aus), Panex, Paralgin (Aus), Pedric, Redutemp, Robigesic (Can), Rounox (Can), Snaplets,

St. Joseph Children's, Supap, Tapanol, Tempra, Tenol, Tylenol, Typap, Valadol, Valorin

Therapeutic Action/Pharmacodynamics: Acetaminophen is a clinically proven analgesic/antipyretic. Acetaminophen produces analgesia by elevation of the pain threshold and antipyresis through action on the hypothalamic heat-regulating center. Acetaminophen is equivalent to aspirin in analgesic and antipyretic effectiveness. Unlike aspirin, acetaminophen has little effect on platelet function, does not affect bleeding time, and generally produces no gastric bleeding. It is unlikely to produce many of the side effects associated with aspirin and aspirin-containing products.

Emergency Uses: Acetaminophen is used as a substitute for aspirin, when the latter is not tolerated or is contraindicated, to reduce fever and/or to temporarily relieve mild to moderate pain. *Adult dose:* 325–650 mg PO every 4–6 hr (maximum 4 g/day); 650 mg PR every 4–6 hr (maximum 4 g/day). *Pediatric dose:* 15 mg/kg every 4–6 hr.

Pharmacokinetics
Absorption: Rapid and almost complete absorption (60–70%) from GI tract; less complete absorption (30–40%) from rectal suppository; peak effect in 1–2 hr; duration is 3–4 hr; half-life is 1–3 hr.
Distribution: Well distributed in all body fluids; crosses placenta.
Metabolism: Extensively metabolized in liver.
Elimination: 90–100% excreted as metabolites in urine; excreted in breast milk.

Contraindications and Precautions: Acetaminophen is contraindicated in patients with hypersensitivity. It is also contraindicated in children under 3 yr, unless directed by a physician; avoid repeated administration to patients with anemia or hepatic disease. Use with caution in arthritic or rheumatoid conditions affecting children under 12 yr; alcoholism; malnutrition; thrombocytopenia.

Adverse/Side Effects: Acute poisoning: CNS: Dizziness, lethargy • GI: Anorexia, nausea, vomiting, epigastric or abdominal pain, diarrhea, onset of hepatotoxicity, hepatic coma, acute renal failure (rare) • Other: Diaphoresis, chills, elevation of serum transaminases (ALT, AST) and bilirubin, hypoglycemia.

Interactions: With chronic coadministration, barbiturates, carbamazepine, phenytoin, and rifampin may increase the potential for chronic hepatotoxicity. Chronic, excessive ingestion of alcohol will increase risk of hepatotoxicity.

Prehospital Considerations
- Individuals with poor nutrition or who have ingested alcohol over prolonged periods are prone to hepato-toxicity even from moderate acetaminophen doses.
- Overdosing and chronic use can cause liver damage and other toxic effects.
- Acetaminophen should not be used for self-medication of pain for more than 10 days in adults or for more than 5 days in children without consulting a physician. It should not be used for fever persisting longer than 3 days and never for fever over 39.5C (103F) or for recurrent fever without medical direction. No more than 5 doses in 24 hr should be given to children unless prescribed by a physician.

ACTIVATED CHARCOAL

Class: Adsorbant

Trade Names: Actidose, Actidose-Aqua, CharcoAid, Charcocaps, Charcodote, InstaChar, LiquiChar, SuperChar

Therapeutic Action/Pharmacodynamics: Activated charcoal is a liquid suspension that adsorbs many drugs and chemicals. It acts by binding (adsorbing) toxic substances, thereby inhibiting their GI adsorption, enterohepatic circulation, and thus bioavailability. It has a tremendous surface area, allowing for a large amount of adsorption; the combined complex formed by the adsorption process is excreted from the body in the feces. It is a general-purpose emergency antidote in the treatment of poisoning by most drugs and chemicals, e.g., acetaminophen, aspirin, atropine, barbiturates, digitalis glycosides, phenytoin, propoxyphene, strychnine, and tricyclic antidepressants, among many others.

Emergency Use: To treat acute ingested poison. *Adult dose:* 1 g/kg mixed with at least 6–8 oz water PO or via nasogastric tube. *Pediatric dose:* Same as adult.

Pharmacokinetics
Absorption: Not absorbed; onset is immediate; peak effect, duration, and half-life are unknown.
Elimination: Excreted in feces.

Contraindications and Precautions: Activated charcoal is contraindicated for treatment of poisonings by cyanide, mineral acids, caustic alkalis, organic solvents, iron, ethanol, and methanol.

Adverse/Side Effects: GI: Vomiting following rapid ingestion of high doses, abdominal cramping, abdominal bloating, constipation (diarrhea from sorbitol additive).

Interactions: May decrease absorption of all other oral medications—administer at least 2 hr apart.

Prehospital Considerations
- Before using charcoal as an antidote, contact medical control or your poison control center for advice.
- Activated charcoal tablets or capsules are less adsorptive and thus less effective than powder or liquid form; therefore, they are not recommended in treatment of acute poisoning.

- Charcoal is most effective when administered as soon as possible after acute poisoning (preferably within 30 min). In an emergency, stir activated charcoal into tap water to make a slurry (about 20–30 g in at least 240 mL of water).
- Activated charcoal can be swallowed or given through a nasogastric tube. If administered too rapidly, your patient may vomit.
- If necessary, taste may be improved by adding a small amount of concentrated fruit juice or chocolate powder to the slurry. Reportedly, these agents do not appreciably alter adsorptive activity.

ADENOSINE

Class: Antidysrhythmic
Trade Name: Adenocard
Therapeutic Action/Pharmacodynamics: Adenosine is a naturally occurring nucleoside that is present in all body cells. Adenosine slows conduction time through the AV node, can interrupt the reentry pathways through the AV and sinoatrial (SA) nodes, and can restore normal sinus rhythm in patients with paroxysmal supraventricular tachycardia (PSVT), including PSVT associated with Wolff-Parkinson-White syndrome. Adenosine is antagonized competitively by methylxanthines such as caffeine and theophylline, and potentiated by blockers of nucleoside transport such as dipyridamole. Its rapid onset and short half-life make adenosine a very safe and effective treatment for PSVT. The usual IV bolus dose of 6 or 12 mg adenosine will have few systemic hemodynamic effects.
Emergency Use: To convert PSVT to a sinus rhythm in patients refractory to common vagal maneuvers. *Adult dose:* 6 mg rapid IV bolus (1–2 sec) followed by a rapid

saline flush; may repeat in 1–2 min at 12 mg. May repeat one more time in 1–2 min at 12 mg. *Pediatric dose:* 0.1 mg/kg rapid IV bolus (1–2 sec) followed by a rapid saline flush; may repeat once in 1–2 min at 0.2 mg/kg. Maximum single dose is 12 mg.

Pharmacokinetics

Absorption: Rapid uptake by erythrocytes and vascular endothelial cells after IV administration; onset and peak effect within 20–30 sec; half-life is 10 sec.

Metabolism: Rapid uptake into cells; degraded by deamination to inosine, hypoxanthine, and adenosine monophosphate.

Elimination: Route of elimination is unknown.

Contraindications and Precautions: Because it slows conduction through the AV junction, adenosine is contraindicated in preexisting second- and third-degree AV block. It may actually produce a short-lasting first-, second-, or third-degree heart block. In extreme cases, transient asystole may occur. Because of the short half-life (10 sec), this usually lasts only a few seconds and resolves without intervention. Do not use in patients with sinus node disease, such as sick sinus syndrome or symptomatic bradycardia, except in patients with a functioning pacemaker. In the presence of atrial flutter or atrial fibrillation, a transient modest slowing of ventricular response may occur immediately following adenosine administration. Adenosine has been administered to a limited number of patients with asthma, and mild to moderate exacerbation of their symptoms has been reported. Respiratory compromise has occurred during adenosine infusion in patients with obstructive pulmonary disease. Adenosine should be used with caution in patients with obstructive lung disease not associated with bronchoconstriction (e.g., emphysema, bronchitis) and should be avoided in patients with bronchoconstriction or bronchospasm (e.g., asthma). Adenosine should be discontinued in any patient who develops severe respiratory difficulties. Never use in patients with a known hypersensitivity to the drug.

Adverse/Side Effects: CV: Facial flushing, headache, sweating, palpitations, atrial fibrillation or flutter, chest pain, hypotension • Respiratory: Shortness of breath/dyspnea, chest pressure, hyperventilation, head pressure • CNS: Lightheadedness, dizziness, tingling in arms, numbness, apprehension, blurred vision, burning sensation, heaviness in arms, neck and back pain • GI: Nausea, metallic taste, tightness in throat, pressure in groin.

Interactions: IV adenosine has been effectively administered in the presence of other cardioactive drugs, such as quinidine, beta-adrenergic blocking agents, calcium channel blocking agents, and angiotensin-converting enzyme inhibitors, without any change in the adverse reaction profile. The effects of adenosine are antagonized by methylxanthines such as caffeine and theophylline. In the presence of these methylxanthines, larger doses of adenosine may be required or adenosine may not be effective. Adenosine effects are potentiated by dipyridamole. Thus, smaller doses of adenosine may be effective in the presence of dipyridamole. Carbamazepine has been reported to increase the degree of heart block produced by other agents. Because the primary effect of adenosine is to decrease conduction through the AV node, higher degrees of heart block may be produced in the presence of carbamazepine.

Prehospital Considerations
- For rapid bolus IV, administer the drug into a large proximal vein and follow with a rapid saline flush.
- The solution must be clear at time of use. Since it contains no preservatives, discard unused portion.

- Monitor ECG, BP, and heart rate every 15–30 sec for several minutes after administration.
- Inform your patient that facial flushing and transient symptoms may occur.

ALBUTEROL

Class: Sympathomimetic bronchodilator

Trade Names: Asmol (Aus), Proventil, Respolin (Aus), Ventolin

Therapeutic Action/Pharacodynamics: Albuterol is a relatively selective beta$_2$ adrenergic stimulant. The prime action of beta-adrenergic drugs is to stimulate adenyl cyclase, the enzyme that catalyzes the formation of cyclic-3′, 5′-adenosine monophosphate (cyclic AMP) from adenosine triphosphate (ATP). The cyclic AMP causes relaxation of the smooth muscles of the bronchial tree, decreasing airway resistance, facilitating mucus drainage, and increasing vital capacity. It exerts minimal effects on beta$_1$ (heart) or alpha (peripheral vasculature) receptors. In therapeutic doses, albuterol, by inhibiting histamine release from mast cells, also reduces the mucus secretion, capillary leaking, and mucosal edema caused by an allergic response in the lungs.

Emergency Uses: To relieve bronchospasm in patients with reversible obstructive airway disease (asthma, chronic bronchitis, emphysema) and acute attacks of bronchospasm. *Adult dose:* 90 mcg via metered-dose inhaler (2 sprays) or 2.5 mg in 2.5–3.0 mL of NS via nebulizer; may repeat as needed. Ventolin is also supplied in Rotacaps for use in a Rotahaler. Two 200-mcg caps should be placed and inhaled. May repeat in 6 hr. *Pediatric dose:* 0.15 mcg/kg in 2.5–3.0 mL of NS via nebulizer; may repeat as needed.

Pharmacokinetics

Absorption: Onset is 5–15 min inhaled; peak effect is 1–1.5 hr; duration is 3–6 hr; half-life is less than 3 hr.
Distribution: When inhaled, albuterol is distributed to muscle cells along the bronchial tree. Very little is systemically absorbed and distributed.
Metabolism: Metabolized in liver; may cross the placenta.
Elimination: 76% of dose eliminated in urine in 3 days.

Contraindications and Precautions: Never use for patients with a known hypersensitivity to the drug.

Adverse/Side Effects: CNS: Tremors, anxiety, dizziness, seizures, headache, insomnia • GI: Nausea, dyspepsia • ENT: Pharyngitis, nasal congestion • CV: Palpitations, tachycardia, hypertension • Respiratory: Bronchospasm, cough, wheezing.

Interactions: Other sympathomimetic aerosol bronchodilators or epinephrine should not be used concomitantly with albuterol. Albuterol should be administered with extreme caution to patients being treated with monoamine oxidase (MAO) inhibitors or tricyclic antidepressants, since the action of albuterol on the vascular system may be potentiated. Beta-receptor blocking agents and albuterol inhibit the effect of each other. Since albuterol may lower serum potassium, care should be taken in patients also using other drugs that lower serum potassium as the effects may be additive.

Prehospital Considerations

- Your patient may be taking albuterol in an oral form. The most common adverse effect associated with oral drug is fine tremor in fingers, which may interfere with precision manual dexterity.
- Expect children 2–6 yr old to be more prone to symptoms of CNS stimulation (hyperactivity, excitement, nervousness, insomnia), tachycardia, and GI symptoms.

Albuterol

11

Rarely do patients receive adequate directions for correct use of their medication and inhaler. Do not assume that they have administered their drug properly.

- Significant subjective improvement in pulmonary function should occur within 60–90 min after drug administration. Reevaluate your patient's condition often and repeat albuterol therapy when indicated.

ALTEPLASE RECOMBINANT (tPA)

Class: Fibrinolytic

Trade Names: Actilyse (Aus), Activase

Therapeutic Action/Pharmacodynamics: This recombinant DNA-derived form of human tissue-type plasminogen activator (tPA) is a fibrinolytic agent. tPA promotes fibrinolysis by forming the active proteolytic enzyme plasmin. Plasmin is capable of degrading fibrin, fibrinogen, and factors V, VIII, and XII.

Emergency Uses: Fibrinolysis in acute myocardial infarction and acute ischemic stroke. *Adult dose:* 15 mg IV, then 0.75 mg/kg (up to 50 mg) over 30 min, then 0.5 mg/kg (up to 35 mg) over 60 min. *Pediatric dose:* Not used.

Fibrinolysis in acute pulmonary embolism. *Adult dose:* 100 mg IV infusion over 2 hr. *Pediatric dose:* Not used.

Pharmacokinetics

Absorption: Onset and peak effects 5–10 min after infusion completed; half-life is 26.5 min.

Metabolism: Metabolized in liver.

Elimination: Excreted in urine.

Contraindications and Precautions: Alteplase is absolutely contraindicated in patients with active internal bleeding, suspected aortic dissection, traumatic CPR (rib fractures, pneumothorax), history of recent hemorrhagic stroke (within 6 months), recent (within 2 months) intracranial or intraspinal surgery or trauma, intracranial tumors, uncontrolled hypertension, pregnancy, or severe allergic reactions to either anistreplase or streptokinase. Use with caution in patients with recent major surgery (within 10 days), cerebral vascular disease, recent GI or GU bleeding, recent trauma, hypertension, age greater than 75, hemorrhagic ophthalmic conditions; use with caution in patients on oral anticoagulants.

Adverse/Side Effects: Hematologic: Internal and superficial bleeding (cerebral, retroperitoneal, GU, GI).

Interactions: Use with caution in patients using other anticoagulant therapy.

Prehospital Considerations
- IV infusion of alteplase should be started as soon as possible after the thrombotic event, preferably within 6 hr for AMI; 3 hr for stroke.
- The 100-mg vial does not contain a vacuum. Follow manufacturer's directions and use supplied transfer device for reconstitution.
- Do not exceed a total dose of 100 mg. Higher doses have been associated with intracranial bleeding.
- Follow infusion of drug by flushing IV tubing with 30–50 mL of NS or D_5W.
- While patient is receiving this medication, do not allow him or her out of bed.
- Check vital signs frequently. Be alert to changes in cardiac rhythm. Dysrhythmias may signal the need to stop therapy.
- Monitor for excess bleeding every 15 min for the first hour of therapy, every 30 min for second to eighth hour, then every 8 hr.
- Monitor neurologic checks throughout drug infusion every 30 min and then every hour thereafter for the first 8 hr after infusion.

- Spontaneous bleeding occurs twice as often with alteplase as with heparin. Protect patient from invasive procedures. IM injections are contraindicated. Also avoid physical manipulation of patient during fibrinolytic therapy to prevent bruising.

AMINOPHYLLINE

Class: Methylxanthine bronchodilator

Trade Names: Aminophylline, Phyllocontin, Somophyllin, Truphyllin

Therapeutic Action/Pharmacodynamics: Methylxanthines cause bronchodilation in a way different from the sympathomimetics. They prolong the effects of beta agonists by blocking the enzyme (phosphodiesterase) that biodegrades them. As a result, the $beta_2$ effects (bronchodilation and decreased mucus secretion) are prolonged. For this reason, they produce mild cardiac and central nervous system stimulation and promote diuresis. Although methylxanthines are primarily used for long-term airway maintenance in COPD, aminophylline may be effective for patients refractory to sympathomimetics and other bronchodilators. Efficacy in acute asthma is controversial. It is not indicated for routine treatment of acute exacerbation of asthma in patients who are receiving optimal therapy with inhaled $beta_2$-adrenergic agonists and steroids.

Emergency Uses: To relieve bronchospasm secondary to asthma or COPD (emphysema, chronic bronchitis). *Adult dose:* 250–500 mg over 20–30 min IV infusion. *Pediatric dose:* 6 mg/kg over 20–30 min; maximum dose should not exceed 12 mg/kg/24 hr.

To relieve bronchospasm in congestive heart failure patients in which additional fluid therapy is contraindicated;

also as a cardiac stimulant and diuretic for patients in congestive heart failure. *Adult dose:* 250–500 mg in 20 mL (via Buretrol or Volutrol container) over 20–30 min IV infusion.

Pharmacokinetics

Absorption: Rapid absorption into bloodstream; onset and peak effect in 15 min; duration varies with age, smoking, and liver function (4–8 hr).
Distribution: Crosses placenta.
Metabolism: Extensively metabolized in liver.
Elimination: Parent drug and metabolites excreted by kidneys; excreted in breast milk.

Contraindications and Precautions: Aminophylline is contraindicated in patients with a hypersensitivity to methylxanthines or patients with uncontrolled cardiac dysrhythmias. Use with extreme caution in patients with cardiac disease or hypertension. Also use with caution in patients with impaired liver function; diabetes mellitus; hyperthyroidism; glaucoma; prostatic hypertrophy; fibro-cystic breast disease; history of peptic ulcer; COPD; acute influenza or in patients receiving influenza immunization; in neonates and young children; and in patients over age 55.

Adverse/Side Effects: CNS: Nervousness, restlessness, depression, insomnia, irritability, headache, dizziness, muscle hyperactivity, convulsions • CV: Cardiac dys-rhythmias, tachycardia, with rapid IV: hyperventilation, chest pain, severe hypotension, cardiac arrest • GI: Nausea, vomiting, anorexia, hematemesis, diarrhea, epigastric pain.

Interactions: In patients with acute exacerbations who are currently taking theophylline-containing preparations (Slo-bid, Theo-dur), serum theophylline levels should be determined prior to the administration of aminophylline, particularly if there are any signs of toxicity. Theophylline preparations interact with many drugs. Cimetidine, erythromycin- and quinolone-class antibiotics can elevate serum theophylline levels.

Prehospital Considerations

- Aminophylline has a very narrow therapeutic range. While administering aminophylline, closely monitor your patient for signs of hypotension, dysrhythmias, and convulsions. A sudden, sharp, unexplained rise in heart rate is a useful clinical indicator of toxicity. Minor symptoms of toxicity often do not precede cardiac arrhythmias or seizures.
- Rapid infusion of IV aminophylline may cause cardiac arrest. Monitor infusion rate carefully.
- Do not use aminophylline solutions if discolored or if crystals are present.
- The elderly, acutely ill, and patients with severe respiratory problems, liver dysfunction, or pulmonary edema are at greater risk of toxicity because of reduced drug clearance.
- Children appear to be more susceptible than adults to the CNS-stimulating effects of methylxanthines (nervousness, restlessness, insomnia, hyperactive reflexes, twitching, convulsions). Dosage reduction may be indicated.
- Smoking (tobacco or marijuana) tends to increase aminophylline elimination (reduces half-life), and therefore dosage requirements may be higher and dosage intervals shorter than in nonsmokers.
- Many popular over-the-counter remedies for treatment of asthma or cough contain ephedrine in combination with various forms of methylxanthines. Always include over-the-counter medications in your history and watch for signs of toxicity.

AMIODARONE

Class: Antidysrhythmic

Trade Names: Aratac (Aus), Cordarone, Cordarone X (Aus), Pacerone

Therapeutic Action/Pharmacodynamics: Amiodarone is unlike other antidysrhythmics in that it acts directly on all cardiac tissues. It is thought to prolong the duration of the action potential and refractory period without significantly affecting the resting membrane potential. The IV formulation relaxes vascular smooth muscle, decreases peripheral vascular resistance, and increases coronary blood flow. Amiodarone also blocks effects of sympathetic stimulation.

Emergency Uses: To treat life-threatening ventricular and supraventricular dysrhythmias, particularly atrial fibrillation. *Adult dose:* 150–300 mg IV over 10 min followed by 1 mg/min over next 6 hr. Maintenance dose is 0.5 mg. The total daily dose should not exceed 2.2 g. Oral loading dose is 800–1,600 mg/day in 1–2 doses, with a maintenance dose of 400–600 mg/day. *Pediatric dose:* 5 mg/kg IV/IO by rapid bolus. Maximum dose is 15 mg/kg. Oral loading dose is 5–15 mg/kg/day divided in 1–2 doses, with a maintenance dose of 5 mg/kg/day.

Pharmacokinetics

Intravenous: Rapid distribution of amiodarone following IV administration, serum concentrations decline to 10% of peak values within 30–45 min. Metabolism and elimination are primarily hepatic. No established relationship between concentration and therapeutic response with short-term IV use. Oral: Oral amiodarone is 50% absorbed. The onset of action is 2–3 days. Peak levels are attained at 3–7 hr. Distribution is widespread and includes adipose tissues, lungs, kidneys, and spleen. Elimination is hepatic and half-life is commonly 40–55 days following oral administration. The drug crosses the placenta and can be found in breast milk.

Contraindications and Precautions: IV amiodarone is contraindicated in patients with a known hypersensitivity to the drug. Because it may decrease automaticity, conductivity, and contractility, do not use IV amiodarone in the presence of cardiogenic shock, severe sinus bradycardia, or advanced AV block unless a pacemaker is available. Oral amiodarone is also contraindicated when episodes of bradycardia have caused syncope except when used in conjunction with a pacemaker. Because it is metabolized in the liver, use with caution in patients with severe liver disease. Also use with caution during pregnancy (category D) and in nursing women.

Adverse/Side Effects: CNS: Peripheral neuropathy (muscle weakness, wasting numbness, tingling), fatigue, abnormal gait, dyskinesias, dizziness, paresthesia, headache. • CV: Bradycardia, hypotension (IV), sinus arrest, cardiogenic shock, CHF, dysrhythmias; AV block • Eye: Corneal microdeposits, optic neuritis, optic neuropathy, blurred vision, permanent blindness, corneal degeneration, macular degeneration, photosensitivity • GI: Anorexia, nausea, vomiting, constipation • Respiratory (pulmonary toxicity): Alveolitis, pneumonitis (fever, dry cough, dyspnea), interstitial pulmonary fibrosis • Skin: Slate-blue pigmentation, photosensitivity, rash • Other (with chronic use): Angioedema, hyperthyroidism or hypothyroidism, hepatotoxicity; may cause neonatal hypo- or hyperthyroidism if taken during pregnancy.

Interactions: Amiodarone significantly increases digoxin levels and enhances pharmacologic effects and toxicities of disopyramide, procainamide, quinidine, flecainide, and lidocaine. It also enhances the anticoagulant effects of oral anticoagulants. Calcium channel blockers and beta blockers may potentiate sinus bradycardia, sinus arrest, or AV block. Amiodarone may increase phenytoin levels 2- to 3-fold. Ritonavir may increase cardiotoxicity. Additional interactions include fentanyl, cyclosporine, cholestyramine, and cimetidine.

Prehospital Considerations

- During IV infusion, carefully monitor blood pressure and slow the infusion if significant hypotension occurs. Bradycardia should be treated by slowing the infusion or discontinuing it if necessary. Sustained monitoring is essential because drug has an unusually long half-life.
- Report adverse reactions promptly. Bear in mind that long elimination half-life means that drug effects will persist long after dosage adjustments are made or drug is discontinued.
- Be alert to signs of pulmonary toxicity: progressive dyspnea, fatigue, cough, pleuritic pain, fever.
- Auscultate chest periodically or when patient complains of respiratory symptoms. Check for diminished breath sounds, rales, pleuritic friction rub; observe breathing pattern. Drug-induced pulmonary function problems must be distinguished from CHF or pneumonia. Keep your medical direction physician informed.
- Monitor heart rate and rhythm and BP until drug response has stabilized. Promptly report symptomatic bradycardia.
- Patients already receiving antidysrhythmic therapy when amiodarone is started must be closely observed for adverse effects, particularly conduction disturbances and exacerbation of dysrhythmias. Dosage of previous agent should be reduced by 30–50% several days after amiodarone therapy is started.

AMRINONE (Inamrinone)

Class: Cardiac inotrope

Trade Name: Inocor

Therapeutic Action/Pharmacodynamics: Amrinone is a class of cardiac inotropic agents with vasodilator activity. It is a phosphodiesterase inhibitor whose mode of action differs from that of the digitalis glycosides and beta-adrenergic stimulants. In patients with depressed myocardial function, it enhances myocardial contractility, increases cardiac output and stroke volume, and reduces right and left ventricular filling pressure, pulmonary capillary wedge pressure (PCWP), and systemic vascular resistance. It is often used when traditional therapies such as digitalis, diuretics, vasodilators, and conventional inotropes have failed for patients with severe congestive heart failure.

Emergency Uses: *Adult dose:* 0.75 mg/kg IV bolus given slowly over 2–3 min, followed by an infusion of 5–15 mg/kg per min. An additional bolus, if needed, can be given in 30 min. Amrinone is used to support cardiac output and systemic vascular resistance in children with septic shock or myocardial dysfunction, such as dilated cardiomyopathy or following cardiac surgery. *Pediatric dose:* 0.75–1.0 mg/kg over 5 min. If the patient tolerates this load, it may be repeated 2 times up to a total load of 3 mg/kg, followed by an infusion of 5–10 mg/kg/min IV.

Pharmacokinetics

Absorption: Onset in 2–5 min; peak effect in 10 min; duration is 0.5–2 hr.

Distribution: Unknown if it crosses placenta or into breast milk.

Metabolism: Metabolized in liver.

Elimination: Excreted primarily in urine.

Contraindications and Precautions: Amrinone is contraindicated in patients with a known hypersensitivity to amrinone or to bisulfites. Use with caution in patients with CHF immediately following acute MI as it may increase myocardial ischemia.

Adverse/Side Effects: CV: Hypotension, dysrhythmias
• GI: Nausea, vomiting, anorexia, abdominal cramps
• Hematologic: Asymptomatic thrombocytopenia (decreased platelets).

Interactions: Amrinone should not be mixed in dextrose- or sodium bicarbonate–containing solutions or administered into an IV line containing furosemide as it may precipitate.

Prehospital Considerations
• Natural color of IV amrinone is clear yellow. Discard discolored solutions and those that contain a precipitate. Store at 15–30C (59–86F) unless otherwise directed. Protect ampules from light.
• During IV administration, monitor BP, heart rate, and respirations and keep your medical direction physician informed. If your patient's BP falls or if dysrhythmias occur, slow or stop the infusion immediately.
• Monitor infusion site to prevent extravasation.
• The chief measurement used to evaluate patient response is relief of symptoms of CHF.
• Amrinone IV preparation contains sodium metabisulfite, a reducing agent to which certain susceptible individuals are allergic. Drug should be discontinued immediately if patient manifests clinical symptoms suggestive of a hypersensitivity reaction.

AMYL NITRITE

Class: Nitrate vasodilator
Trade Name: Amyl Nitrite
Therapeutic Action/Pharmacodynamics: Amyl nitrite is a short-acting vasodilator and smooth muscle relaxant

with actions, contraindications, and adverse reactions similar to those of nitroglycerin. Its action in the treatment of cyanide poisoning is based on the ability of amyl nitrite to convert hemoglobin to methemoglobin, which forms a nontoxic complex with the cyanide ion to form cyanomethemoglobin, which can be enzymatically degraded. Amyl nitrite is supplied in a glass ampule that is broken and its contents immediately inhaled.

Emergency Use: As the initial adjunct antidote in the treatment of cyanide poisoning. *Adult dose:* 0.3-mL ampule crushed every minute and inhaled for 15–30 sec until sodium nitrite infusion is ready. *Pediatric dose:* Same as for adult.

Pharmacokinetics

Absorption: Rapidly absorbed from mucous membranes; onset is 10–30 sec; peak effect is unknown; duration is 3–5 min.

Contraindications and Precautions: There are no contraindications to the use of amyl nitrite in the management of acute cyanide poisoning.

Adverse/Side Effects: CNS: Headache, dizziness, weakness, syncope • CV: Transient flushing, orthostatic hypotension, palpitations, cardiovascular collapse, tachycardia • Respiratory: Respiratory depression • GI: Nausea, vomiting.

Interactions: The hypotensive effects of amyl nitrite may be potentiated by antihypertensive agents, beta blockers, calcium channel blockers, and certain antiemetics (phenothiazines).

Prehospital Considerations

- To prepare for administration, wrap the ampule in gauze or cloth and crush between your fingers.
- Syncope, due to a sudden drop in systolic BP, sometimes follows amyl nitrite inhalation, particularly in the elderly. Patient should be sitting while and immediately after drug is administered.

- Amyl nitrite is volatile and highly flammable. When mixed with air or oxygen, it forms a mixture that can explode if ignited.
- After administration of drug, note length of time required for pain to subside; monitor vital signs until they are stable. Rapid pulse, which usually lasts for a brief period, is an expected baroreceptor response to the fall in BP produced by the nitrite ion.
- Inform patient that drug has a strong, unpleasant odor (often compared to an athletic locker room).
- Amyl nitrite is a drug of abuse and should be kept in a secure place with your narcotics.

ANISTREPLASE (APSAC)

Class: Fibrinolytic

Trade Name: Eminase

Therapeutic Action/Pharmacodynamics: Anisoylated plasminogen-streptokinase activator complex (APSAC) causes fibrinolysis (dissolution of a clot) by converting plasminogen (present in the blood) to plasmin. Plasmin then digests fibrin and fibrinogen, causing the blood clot to dissolve.

Emergency Use: To reduce infarct size in acute MI by fibrinolysis. *Adult dose:* 30 units IV push over 2–5 min.

Pharmacokinetics

Absorption: Immediate onset; peak effect in 45 min; duration is 6 hr to 2 days; half-life is 105–120 min.

Metabolism: Metabolized in plasma.

Contraindications and Precautions: APSAC is absolutely contraindicated in patients with active internal bleeding, suspected aortic dissection, traumatic CPR (rib fractures, pneumothorax), history of recent stroke (within 6 months), recent (within 2 months) intracranial or intraspinal surgery or trauma, intracranial tumors, uncontrolled hypertension, pregnancy, or severe allergic reactions to either anistreplase or streptokinase. Use with caution in patients with recent major surgery (within 10 days), cerebral vascular disease, pregnancy, recent GI or GU bleeding, recent trauma, hypertension, hemorrhagic ophthalmic conditions, and current use of oral anticoagulants, and in those over age 75.

Adverse/Side Effects: CV: Hemorrhage, reperfusion dysrhythmias, hypotension • Hypersensitivity: Anaphylactic and anaphylactoid reactions in less than 1% of patients.

Interactions: Use with caution in patients on anticoagulant therapy.

Prehospital Considerations
- The drug should be administered as soon as possible following the onset of clinical symptoms of acute MI.
- Dilute each dose with 5 mL sterile water for injection. Slowly add diluent, rolling vial to mix; do not shake. Do not further dilute reconstituted solution, and discard if it is not used within 30 min.
- Inject over 2–5 min directly into vein or IV line through the most proximal port.
- During administration, only essential handling or moving of the patient should be done.
- Diluted solution may be clear to pale yellow. Do not administer if particulate matter is present.
- Spontaneous bleeding occurs twice as often with anistreplase as with heparin. Protect patient from invasive procedures: IM injections are contraindicated. Also prevent manipulation during fibrinolytic therapy to prevent bruising.
- Report signs of bleeding: gum bleeding, epistaxis, hematoma, spontaneous ecchymosis, oozing at catheter site, increased pain from internal bleeding.

The anistreplase infusion should be interrupted, then resumed when bleeding stops.

- APSAC may be ineffective if given within 1 yr of prior streptokinase or APSAC therapy.
- Be prepared to resuscitate your patient if anaphylaxis or reperfusion dysrhythmias occur.

ASPIRIN (Acetylsalicylic Acid)

Classes: Analgesic; antipyretic; nonsteroidal anti-inflammatory drug; platelet inhibitor

Trade Names: Alka-Seltzer, A.S.A., Aspergum, Aspro (Aus), Astrin (Can), Bayer, Bext (Aus), Corhyphen (Can), Cosprin, Easprin, Ecotrin, Empirin, Entrophen (Can), Halfprin, Measurin, Novasen (Can), St. Joseph Children's, Solprin (Aus), Supasa (Aus), Triaphen-10, Vincent's Powders (Aus), Winsprin Capules (Aus), ZORprin.

Therapeutic Action/Pharmacodynamics: Aspirin is an anti-inflammatory agent and an inhibitor of platelet function. The major actions of aspirin appear to be associated primarily with inhibiting the formation of prostaglandins involved in the production of inflammation, pain, and fever. As an anti-inflammatory agent, aspirin appears to be involved in reducing the spread of inflammation by inhibiting prostaglandin synthesis. These anti-inflammatory actions also contribute to analgesic effects. As an analgesic, it relieves mild to moderate pain by acting on the peripheral nervous system with limited action in the central nervous system (hypothalamus). In addition to inhibiting prostaglandin synthesis, aspirin lowers body temperature in fever by indirectly causing centrally mediated peripheral vasodilation and sweating. As an antiplatelet agent, aspirin (but not other salicylates) powerfully inhibits platelet aggregation by blocking the formation of thromboxane A_2, which causes platelets to aggregate and arteries to constrict. This action results in an overall reduction in mortality associated with myocardial infarction. It also reduces the rate of reinfarction and stroke.

Emergency Uses: To inhibit clot formation in the presence of chest pain suggestive of an acute myocardial infarction. To inhibit clot formation associated with thrombotic stroke. *Adult dose:* 160–325 mg PO (chewable).

Pharmacokinetics

Absorption: 80–100% absorbed (depending on formulation), primarily in stomach and upper small intestine; onset is 5–30 min; peak levels in 15 min to 2 hr; duration is 1–4 hr; half-life is 15–20 min.

Distribution: Widely distributed in most body tissues; crosses placenta.

Metabolism: Aspirin is hydrolyzed to salicylate in GI mucosa, plasma, and erythrocytes; salicylate is metabolized in liver.

Elimination: 50% of dose is eliminated in the urine in 2–4 hr. Excreted in breast milk.

Contraindications and Precautions: Aspirin is contraindicated in patients with a history of hypersensitivity to salicylates including methyl salicylate (oil of wintergreen), active ulcer disease, and asthma. It should be used with caution in patients with allergies to other NSAIDS, and in those who have other bleeding disorders. Because of the possible association of aspirin usage with Reye's syndrome, do not give aspirin to children or teenagers with symptoms of varicella (chickenpox) or influenza-like illnesses before consulting a physician.

Adverse/Side Effects: CNS: Dizziness, confusion, drowsiness • ENT: Tinnitus, hearing loss • GI: Nausea, vomiting, diarrhea, anorexia, heartburn, stomach pains,

ulceration, occult bleeding, GI bleeding• Hematologic:
Thrombocytopenia, hemolytic anemia• Hypersensitivity:
Urticaria, bronchospasm, anaphylactic shock, laryngeal
edema• Skin: Petechiae, easy bruising, rash • Other:
Impaired renal function, prolonged bleeding time, pro-
longed pregnancy and labor with increased bleeding.

Interactions: Anticoagulants increase risk of bleeding.
Oral hypoglycemic agents increase hypoglycemic activity
with aspirin doses greater than 2 g/day.

Prehospital Considerations

- Baby aspirin is preferred in the emergency setting
  because it can be chewed and swallowed, and it is more
  palatable to the nauseated MI patient. Administer 2
  tablets (81 mg each) as soon as possible when indicated.
- Gastric irritation may be minimized by administering
  with a full glass of water (240 mL), or with milk, food,
  or antacid. Enteric-coated tablets dissolve too quickly if
  administered with milk; also they should not be crushed
  or chewed.
- In adults, a sensation of fullness in the ears, tinnitus,
  and decreased or muffled hearing are the most frequent
  symptoms associated with chronic salicylate overdosage.
- Potential for toxicity is high in elderly chronic aspirin
  users because they have less serum protein to bind salicylate and also are less able to excrete it.
- Children tend to manifest salicylate toxicity by hyperventilation, agitation, mental confusion, or other behavioral
  changes, drowsiness, lethargy, sweating, and constipation.
- In children, and infants particularly, salicylate toxicity is
  enhanced by the dehydration that frequently accom-
  panies fever or illness. Monitor these patients closely.
- Buffered aspirin preparations in an effervescent vehicle,
  e.g., Alka-Seltzer, are more rapidly absorbed than plain
  aspirin and reportedly cause less GI irritation and
  bleeding. Alka-Seltzer, however, has a high sodium

Aspirin

content (approximately 24 mEq of sodium per 32-mg tablet).

- Buffered aspirin or aspirin administered with an antacid may be better tolerated than conventional tablets.
- Discontinue use with onset of ringing or buzzing in the ears, impaired hearing, dizziness, or GI discomfort or bleeding, and report to physician. Hearing impairment resulting from salicylate overdosage can generally be reversed within 24 hr by reducing the dose.
- Avoid other medications containing aspirin unless directed by physician, because of danger of overdosing. (There are more than 500 OTC aspirin-containing compounds.)

ATENOLOL

Classes: Antidysrhythmic; antihypertensive

Trade Names: Apo-Atenolol (Can), Tenormin

Therapeutic Action/Pharmacodynamics: Atenolol is a beta-blocking agent selective for beta$_1$-adrenergic receptors located chiefly in cardiac muscle. With large doses, the selectivity for beta$_1$-adrenergic receptors is lost, and inhibition of beta$_2$-adrenergic receptors may lead to increased airway resistance, especially in patients with asthma and COPD. Cardiac effects are primarily due to competitive inhibition of catecholamine binding at beta-adrenergic receptor sites. Atenolol reduces the rate and force of cardiac contraction (negative inotropic action); cardiac output and blood pressure are reduced. Atenolol increases peripheral vascular resistance.

Emergency Uses: To treat acute coronary syndromes, including non-Q-wave MI and unstable angina. Beta blockers also reduce the incidence of ventricular fibrillation. *Adult dose:* 5 mg slow IV (over 5 min); wait 10 min, then if the first dose is well tolerated, give a second 5-mg slow IV (over 5 min). *Pediatric dose:* 0.8–1.5 mg/kg/day PO (maximum 2 mg/kg/day).

Pharmacokinetics

Absorption: 50% of oral dose absorbed; peak effect in 2–4 hr PO, 5 min IV; duration of effect is 24 hr; half-life is 6–7 hr.
Distribution: Does not readily cross blood-brain barrier.
Metabolism: No hepatic metabolism.
Elimination: 40–50% excreted in urine, 50–60% in feces.

Contraindications and Precautions: Atenolol is contraindicated in sinus bradycardia, greater than first-degree heart block, CHF, cardiogenic shock. Use caution in asthma, COPD, and CHF controlled by digitalis and diuretics. Safe use during pregnancy (category C), in nursing women, and in children is not established.

Adverse/Side Effects: CNS: Dizziness, vertigo, light-headedness, syncope, fatigue or weakness, lethargy, drowsiness, insomnia, depression • CV: Bradycardia, hypotension, CHF, cold extremities, leg pains, dysrhythmias • GI: Nausea, vomiting, diarrhea • Respiratory: Pulmonary edema, dyspnea, bronchospasm • Other: May mask symptoms of hypoglycemia.

Interactions: Atropine and other anticholinergics can increase atenolol absorption from the GI tract; NSAIDs can decrease hypotensive effects. May mask symptoms of hypoglycemia induced by insulin and sulfonylureas. May increase lidocaine levels and toxicity; pharmacologic effects of atenolol and verapamil are increased when used concomitantly.

Prehospital Considerations

- IV atenolol is given no faster than 1 mg/min (5 mg/5 min).
- IV atenolol may be diluted in up to 50 mL of D_5W or NS.

Atenolol

- Store in tightly covered, light-resistant containers at 15–30C (59–86F) unless otherwise directed.
- ECG monitoring is essential because of the possibility of drug-induced arrhythmias.
- Instruct patient to report immediately any increased dyspnea or decreased exercise tolerance.
- Monitor pulse, blood pressure, ECG, and respirations throughout therapy.

ATRACURIUM

Class: Nondepolarizing neuromuscular blocker

Trade Name: Tracrium

Therapeutic Action/Pharmacodynamics: Atracurium is a synthetic skeletal muscle relaxant pharmacologically similar to tubocurarine that produces shorter duration of neuromuscular blockade, exhibits minimal direct effects on cardiovascular system, and has less histamine-releasing action. It has minimal cumulative tendency with subsequent doses if recovery from the drug begins before dose is repeated. It inhibits neuromuscular transmission by binding competitively with acetylcholine to muscle end-plate receptors. Atracurium lacks analgesic action and has no apparent effect on pain threshold, consciousness, or cerebration.

Emergency Uses: To produce skeletal muscle relaxation to facilitate endotracheal intubation and positive pressure ventilation. *Adult dose:* 0.4–0.5 mg/kg IV. *Pediatric dose:* less than 2 yr: 0.3–0.4 mg/kg IV; more than 2 yr: same as for adult.

Pharmacokinetics

Absorption: Onset is 2 min; peak effect is 3–5 min, duration is 35–70 min; half-life is 20 min.

Distribution: Well distributed to tissues and extracellular fluids; crosses placenta.

Metabolism: Rapid nonenzymatic degradation in bloodstream.
Elimination: 70–90% excreted in urine within 5–7 hr.

Contraindications and Precautions: Atracurium is contraindicated in myasthenia gravis. It should be used with caution when appreciable histamine release would be hazardous (as in asthma or anaphylactoid reactions, significant cardiovascular disease).

Adverse/Side Effects: CV: Bradycardia, tachycardia • Respiratory: Respiratory depression • Other: Increased salivation, anaphylaxis.

Interactions: Neuromuscular blockade may be enhanced in the presence of the following drugs: aminoglycosides, bacitracin, polymyxin B, clindamycin, lidocaine, parenteral magnesium, quinidine, quinine, trimethaphan, verapamil, diuretics, lithium, and succinylcholine. Narcotic analgesics may present the possibility of additive respiratory depression. Phenytoin may cause resistance to or reversal of neuromuscular blockade. Atracurium is incompatible with alkaline solutions (e.g., barbiturates, sodium bicarbonate). Do not mix in same syringe or administer through same needle as used for alkaline solutions. Reportedly compatible with 5% dextrose and 0.9% NaCl.

Prehospital Considerations
- Equipment required for endotracheal intubation, administration of oxygen under positive pressure, artificial respiration, and assisted or controlled ventilation should be immediately available.
- Monitor BP, pulse, and respirations and evaluate your patient's recovery from neuromuscular blocking (curare-like) effect as evidenced by ability to breathe naturally or to take deep breaths and cough, keep eyes open, lift head keeping mouth closed, adequacy of hand-grip strength.

Atracurium

- Patient may find oral communication difficult until head and neck muscles recover from blockade effects.
- Recovery from neuromuscular blockade usually begins 35–45 min after drug administration and is almost complete in about 1 hr. Note that recovery time may be delayed in patients with cardiovascular disease, edematous states, and in the elderly.

ATROPINE

Class: Parasympatholytic

Trade Name: Atropine

Therapeutic Action/Pharmacodynamics: Atropine exerts its effects on the autonomic nervous system. It is a competitive antagonist that selectively blocks all muscarinic responses to acetylcholine (ACh). By blocking vagal (parasympathetic) impulses to the heart, it increases SA node discharge, enhances conduction through the AV junction, and increases cardiac output. Its antisecretory action suppresses sweating, lacrimation, salivation, and secretions from the upper and lower respiratory tract. Atropine is a potent bronchodilator when bronchoconstriction has been induced by parasympathomimetics. Produces mydriasis (dilation of pupils) and cycloplegia (paralysis of accommodation) by blocking responses of iris sphincter muscle and ciliary muscle of lens to cholinergic stimulation.

Emergency Uses: To increase cardiac output in symptomatic bradycardia (e.g., altered mental status, hypotension, cardiac ectopy, chest pain, CHF). *Adult dose:* 0.5–1.0 mg IV, 2 mg ET. May repeat every 3–5 min up to 3.0 mg. *Pediatric dose:* 0.02 mg/kg IV, 0.04 mg/kg ET. Minimum dose is 0.1 mg. May repeat in 5 min up to 1 mg.

To restore cardiac function in bradyasystolic cardiac arrest. *Adult dose:* 1 mg IV, 2 mg ET. May repeat every 3–5 min up to 3.0 mg. *Pediatric dose:* Not used in pediatric asystole.

As a parasympatholytic in organophosphate poisoning. *Adult dose:* 2–5 mg IV/IM every 10–15 min. *Pediatric dose:* 0.05 mg/kg IV/IM/IO every 10–15 min.

Pharmacokinetics

Absorption: Atropine is well absorbed from all administration sites; peak effect is 20–60 min IM, 2–4 min IV; duration is 4 hr; half-life is 2–3 hr.

Distribution: Distributed in most body tissues; crosses blood-brain barrier and placenta.

Metabolism: Metabolized in liver.

Elimination: 77–94% excreted in urine in 24 hr.

Contraindications and Precautions: No contraindications in the emergency setting. Use with caution in patients with signs and symptoms of acute myocardial ischemia or infarction. Because it raises intraocular pressure, use with caution in patients with glaucoma.

Adverse/Side Effects: CNS: Headache, ataxia, dizziness, excitement, irritability, convulsions, drowsiness, fatigue, weakness; mental depression, confusion, disorientation, hallucinations • CV: Hypertension or hypotension, ventricular tachycardia, palpitations, paradoxical bradycardia, AV dissociation, atrial or ventricular fibrillation • Eye: Mydriasis, blurred vision, photophobia, increased intraocular pressure, cycloplegia, eye dryness, local redness • GI: Dry mouth with thirst, dysphagia, loss of taste; nausea, vomiting, constipation, delayed gastric emptying • GU: Urinary hesitancy and retention, dysuria, impotence • Skin: Flushed, dry skin; anhydrosis, rash, urticaria, contact dermatitis, allergic conjunctivitis.

Atropine

Interactions: Amantadine, antihistamines, tricyclic anti-depressants, quinidine, disopyramide, procainamide can add to the anticholinergic effects of atropine. Levodopa effects are decreased. Methotrimeptrazine may precipitate extrapyramidal effects. Phenothiazines' antipsychotic effects are decreased (decreased absorption).

Prehospital Considerations
- Smaller doses of atropine are indicated for the elderly.
- Monitor vital signs $ETCO_2$. Pulse is a sensitive indicator of patient's response to atropine. Be alert to changes in quality, rate, and rhythm of pulse and respiration and to changes in blood pressure and temperature.
- Initial paradoxic bradycardia following IV atropine usually lasts only 1–2 min; it most likely occurs when IV is administered slowly (more than 1 min) or when small doses (less than 0.5 mg) are used.
- Atropine may actually worsen the bradycardia associated with Mobitz II and complete AV block. In these cases, use transcutaneous pacing.
- Always rule out hypoxia as the cause for bradycardia in infants and small children. Atropine is indicated only after oxygen and epinephrine fail.

BRETYLIUM

Class: Antidysrhythmic

Trade Names: Bretylate (Aus), Bretylol

Therapeutic Action/Pharmacodynamics: The mechanism of action of bretylium is complex and not fully understood. It suppresses ventricular fibrillation by direct action on the myocardium and ventricular tachycardia by adrenergic blockade. Shortly after administration, norepinephrine is released from adrenergic postganglionic nerve terminals, resulting in a moderate increase in BP, heart rate, and ventricular irritability. Subsequently, drug-induced release and reuptake of norepinephrine are blocked, leading to a state resembling surgical sympathectomy. Bretylium suppresses ventricular tachydysrhythmias with a reentry mechanism, elevates the fibrillation threshold, and decreases ectopic foci without changing PR, QT, and QRS intervals. Orthostatic hypotension occurs commonly as a result of peripheral adrenergic blockade; some degree of hypotension may occur even while your patient is supine. Tolerance to this effect develops after several days in most patients as adrenergic receptors become more responsive to circulating catecholamines. Because onset of desired action is delayed, bretylium is not a first-line antidysrhythmic agent.

Emergency Uses: To treat ventricular tachycardia and ventricular fibrillation refractory to lidocaine. *Adult dose:* 5 mg/kg IV; repeat at 10 mg/kg IV every 15–30 min up to 30 mg/kg. Following conversion, administer IV infusion at 1–2 mg/min. *Pediatric dose:* 5 mg/kg IV; repeat bolus of 10 mg/kg in 15–30 min.

Pharmacodynamics
Absorption: Onset and peak effect are minutes after IV; duration is 6–24 hr; half-life is 4–17 hr.
Distribution: Does not cross blood-brain barrier; not known if it crosses placenta or is distributed into breast milk.
Metabolism: Not metabolized.
Elimination: 70–80% excreted in urine in 24 hr.

Contraindications and Precautions: There are no contraindications when used in life-threatening refractory ventricular dysrhythmias. Safe use in pregnancy (category C), in nursing mothers, and in children is not established. Use with caution in patients with digitalis-induced dysrhythmias; fixed cardiac output, e.g., severe aortic stenosis or severe pulmonary hypertension (profound hypotension can result without compensatory increase in cardiac output); sinus bradycardia; angina pectoris; or impaired renal function; and in patients on digitalis maintenance.

Adverse/Side Effects: CV: Both supine and postural hypotension with dizziness, vertigo, light-headedness, faintness, syncope, transitory hypertension, bradycardia, increased frequency of PVCs, exacerbation of digitalis-induced dysrhythmias • GI: Nausea, vomiting (particularly with rapid IV) • Other: Respiratory depression.

Interactions: Bretylium can interact with other antidysrhythmic drugs (procainamide, quinidine, disopyramide, propranolol, lidocaine), causing either antagonistic or additive effects. Antihypertensive agents will add to hypotensive effects. The initial release of norepinephrine may cause the worsening of digitalis-induced dysrhythmias.

Prehospital Considerations
- Anticipate vomiting. IV administration is associated with a high incidence of nausea and vomiting. These side effects can be minimized by slow administration of drug (10 min or more).
- Establish baseline readings and monitor BP and ECG when drug is administered. Observe for initial transient rise in BP, increased heart rate, PVCs and other dysrhythmias, or worsening of existing dysrhythmias, which may occur within a few minutes to 1 hr after drug administration.
- Initial effect of hypertension is usually followed within 1 hr by a fall in supine BP and by orthostatic hypotension.
- Bretylium has been removed from ACLS algorithms and guidelines because of a high incidence of side effects, the availability of safer agents, and the limited availability and supply of the drug.

BUMETANIDE

Class: Loop diuretic

Trade Names: Bumex, Burinex (Aus)

Therapeutic Action/Pharmacodynamics: Bumetanide is a sulfonamide derivative structurally related to furosemide and with similar pharmacologic effects. It features a more rapid rate of onset, a more potent diuretic effect (40 times greater), and a shorter duration of action than that of furosemide. Bumetanide inhibits sodium and chloride reabsorption by direct action on proximal ascending limb of the loop of Henle. It also appears to inhibit phosphate and bicarbonate reabsorption. At usual diuretic doses, it produces only mild hypotensive effects. Causes both potassium and magnesium wastage.

Emergency Uses: To promote diuresis in congestive heart failure and pulmonary edema. *Adult dose:* 0.5–1 mg IM/IV over 1–2 min. Repeat doses may be administered in 2–3 hr as needed.

Pharmacokinetics
Absorption: IV onset is rapid; peak effect in 15–30 min; duration is 3.5–4.0 hr; half-life is 60–90 min.
Distribution: Distributed into breast milk.
Metabolism: Partially metabolized in liver.
Elimination: 80% excreted in urine in 48 hr, 10–20% excreted in feces.

Contraindications and Precautions: Bumetanide is contraindicated in patients with known hypersensitivity to bumetanide or to other sulfonamides. Its use in pregnancy should be limited to life-threatening situations in which the benefits of using bumetanide outweigh the risks.

Adverse/Side Effects: CNS: Dizziness, headache, weakness, fatigue • CV: Hypotension, ECG changes, chest pain, hypovolemia • GI: Nausea, vomiting, abdominal or

stomach pain, GI distress, diarrhea, dry mouth
• Musculoskeletal: Muscle cramps, muscle pain, stiffness or tenderness; arthritic pain • Ototoxicity: Ear discomfort, ringing or buzzing in ears, impaired hearing • Other: Sweating, hyperventilation.

Interactions: Bumetanide increases the risk of hypokalemia-induced digoxin toxicity; NSAIDs may attenuate diuretic and hypotensive response; probenecid may antagonize diuretic activity; bumetanide may decrease renal elimination of lithium.

Prehospital Considerations

- Drug will discolor on exposure to light. Inspect parenteral bumetanide before administration. Discard if it contains particles or is discolored.
- Store in tight, light-resistant container at 15–30C (59–86F) unless otherwise directed.
- Monitor BP and pulse rate. Assess for hypovolemia by assessing BP and pulse rate while patient is lying, sitting, and standing.
- High doses or frequent administration, particularly in the elderly, can cause profound diuresis, hypovolemia, and resulting circulatory collapse with development of thrombi and emboli. Careful monitoring is essential.
- Patients with hepatic disease should be carefully observed. Alterations in fluid and electrolyte balance can precipitate encephalopathy (inappropriate behavior, altered mood, impaired judgment, confusion, drowsiness, coma).

BUTORPHANOL

Class: Synthetic narcotic (opiate) analgesic
Trade Name: Stadol
Therapeutic Action/Pharmacodynamics: Butorphanol is a synthetic, centrally acting analgesic with mixed narcotic

agonist and antagonist actions. It acts as an agonist on one type of opioid receptor and as a competitive antagonist on others. The site of analgesic action is believed to be sub-cortical, possibly in the limbic system. On a weight basis, analgesic potency appears to be about 5 times that of morphine, 40 times that of meperidine, and 15–30 times that of pentazocine. Its narcotic antagonist potential is approximately 30 times that of pentazocine and 1/40 that of naloxone. Two mg of butorphanol produce about the same degree of respiratory depression as 10 mg of morphine. Respiratory depression does not increase appreciably with higher doses, as it does with morphine, but duration of action increases. Like pentazocine, analgesic doses may increase pulmonary arterial pressure and cardiac workload. Butorphanol appears to have some potential for dependence. It tends to inhibit release of antidiuretic hormone (ADH) from posterior pituitary. It is a Schedule IV narcotic.

Emergency Use: To relieve moderate to severe pain. *Adult dose:* 1 mg IV or 3–4 mg IM every 3–4 hr as needed.

Pharmacokinetics
Absorption: Onset is 10–15 min IM, 2–3 min IV; peak effect is 0.5–1.0 hr IM, 4–5 min IV; duration is 3–4 hr IM/IV; half-life is 3–4 hr.
Distribution: Crosses placenta; distributed into breast milk.
Metabolism: Metabolized in liver in inactive metabolites.
Elimination: Excreted primarily in urine.

Contraindications and Precautions: Butorphanol is contraindicated in patients with a known hypersensitivity to the drug. Since it may act as a narcotic antagonist and produce withdrawal symptoms, use it with caution in narcotic-dependent patients. Safe use during pregnancy prior to labor (category C), in nursing mothers, and in children under 18 yr has not been established. Do not use butorphanol in the presence of a head injury or undiagnosed abdominal pain as it will mask the symptoms before a diagnosis can be confirmed. This drug can also cause an increase in cerebrospinal pressure.

Adverse/Side Effects: CNS: Drowsiness, sedation, headache, vertigo, dizziness, floating feeling, weakness, lethargy, confusion, light-headedness, insomnia, nervousness • Respiratory: Respiratory depression • CV: Palpitation, bradycardia • GI: Nausea • Skin: Clammy skin, tingling sensation, flushing and warmth, cyanosis of extremities, diaphoresis, sensitivity to cold, urticaria, pruritus.

Interactions: Alcohol and other CNS depressants augment CNS and respiratory depression.

Prehospital Considerations
- Since the effects are unpredictable in older patients, consider reducing the dose and administering smaller repeated doses rather than one large bolus.
- Store at 15–30C (59–86F) unless otherwise directed. Protect from light.
- Monitor for respiratory depression. Do not administer drug if respiratory rate is less than 12 breaths/min. If respirations decrease, you may reverse the effects of butorphanol with naloxone.
- Monitor vital signs. Report marked changes in BP or bradycardia.
- Butorphanol has habit-forming potential.
- Because butorphanol has agonist as well as antagonist actions, it can induce acute withdrawal symptoms in opiate-dependent patients.
- Because of its potential for abuse, butorphanol should be secured and inventoried daily.

Butorphanol

CALCIUM CHLORIDE

Class: Electrolyte

Trade Names: Calciject (Aus), Calcium Chloride

Therapeutic Action/Pharmacodynamics: Calcium chloride provides elemental calcium in the form of the cation Ca^{++}. Calcium is necessary for many physiologic activities. It is an essential element for regulating the excitation threshold of nerves and muscles, for blood-clotting mechanisms, maintenance of renal function, for body skeleton and teeth. Calcium causes a significant increase in myocardial contractility and in ventricular automaticity. It also plays a role in regulating the storage and release of neurotransmitters and hormones; regulating amino acid uptake and absorption of vitamin B_{12}; gastrin secretion, and in maintaining structural and functional integrity of cell membranes and capillaries. Its excess chloride ions promote acidosis and temporary (1–2 days) diuresis secondary to the excretion of sodium. It is used as an antidote for some electrolyte imbalances, for magnesium sulfate overdose, and to minimize the side effects from calcium channel blocker usage. The actions of calcium chloride are similar to those of calcium gluconate, but since it ionizes more readily, it is more potent than calcium gluconate and more irritating to tissues.

Emergency Uses: To treat hyperkalemia (elevated potassium), hypocalcemia (decreased calcium), hypermagnesemia (elevated magnesium), and calcium channel blocker toxicity. *Adult dose:* 2–4 mg/kg (10% solution) IV every 10 min as needed. *Pediatric dose:* 20 mg/kg (10% solution) IV, repeated once in 10 min as needed.

Pharmacokinetics

Absorption: Onset and peak effects are immediate; duration is unknown.
Distribution: Crosses placenta.

Elimination: Primarily excreted in feces; small amounts excreted in urine, pancreatic juice, saliva, and breast milk.

Contraindications and Precautions: Calcium chloride is contraindicated in ventricular fibrillation, hypercalcemia, and possible digitalis toxicity. It should be used with caution in patients taking digoxin as it may precipitate toxicity. Safe use during pregnancy prior to labor (category C), in nursing mothers, and in children is not established.

Adverse/Side Effects: CNS: Tingling sensation, fainting • Skin: Sensations of heat waves (peripheral vasodilation), pain and burning at IV site with rapid IV, necrosis and sloughing (with extravasation) • CV: Hypotension, bradycardia, cardiac dysrhythmias, cardiac arrest, severe venous thrombosis.

Interactions: Calcium chloride will interact with sodium bicarbonate and form a precipitate. It may enhance inotropic and toxic effects of digoxin and antagonize the effects of verapamil and possibly other calcium channel blockers.

Prehospital Considerations

- Extravasation must be avoided during IV injection, since cellulitis, necrosis, and sloughing can result. Give at 0.5–1.0 mL/min or more slowly if irritation develops. Use a small-bore needle and inject into a large vein to minimize venous irritation and undesirable reactions. If given IV to children, scalp veins should be avoided.
- IV injection may be accompanied by cutaneous burning sensation and peripheral vasodilation, with moderate fall in BP. Monitor ECG, BP, and flow rate and observe patient closely during administration.
- Always flush your IV line prior to and immediately following administration of drugs such as sodium bicarbonate or catecholamines to avoid forming a precipitate.

CALCIUM GLUCONATE

Class: Electrolyte

Trade Name: Kalcinate

Therapeutic Action/Pharmacodynamics: Calcium gluconate provides elemental calcium in the form of the cation Ca^{++}. Calcium is necessary for many physiologic activities. It is an essential element for regulating the excitation threshold of nerves and muscles, for blood-clotting mechanisms, for maintenance of renal function, and for the development of skeletal bones and teeth. Calcium causes a significant increase in myocardial contractility and in ventricular automaticity. It also plays a role in regulating the storage and release of neurotransmitters and hormones; regulating amino acid uptake and absorption of vitamin B_{12}; controlling gastrin secretion; and maintaining structural and functional integrity of cell membranes and capillaries. Calcium gluconate acts like digitalis on the heart, increasing cardiac muscle tone and force of systolic contractions (positive inotropic effect), making it especially useful for patients with sympathetic blockade.

Emergency Uses: To treat cardiac toxicity of hyperkalemia, as an antidote for hypermagnesemia, and to treat calcium channel blocker overdose. *Adult dose:* 5–8 mL of a 10% solution. Repeat as necessary at 10-min intervals.

Pharmacokinetics

Absorption: Onset and peak effects are immediate; duration is unknown.

Distribution: Crosses placenta.

Elimination: Primarily excreted in feces; small amounts excreted in urine, pancreatic juice, saliva, and breast milk.

Contraindications and Precautions: Calcium gluconate is contraindicated in ventricular fibrillation. Use with caution in digitalized patients, renal or cardiac insufficiency, and immobilized patients.

Adverse/Side Effects: CNS: Tingling sensations • CV: Hypotension, bradycardia and other dysrhythmias, syncope, cardiac arrest • Local reactions: Tissue irritation, burning, cellulitis, soft tissue calcification, necrosis, and sloughing (following IV extravasation).

Interactions: Calcium gluconate will interact with sodium bicarbonate and form a precipitate. It may enhance inotropic and toxic effects of digoxin and antagonize the effects of verapamil and possibly other calcium channel blockers.

Prehospital Considerations

- IV calcium should be administered slowly through a small-bore needle into a large vein to avoid possibility of extravasation and resultant necrosis. If calcium is administered to children, scalp veins should be avoided.
- High concentrations of calcium suddenly reaching the heart can cause fatal cardiac arrest.
- Direct IV injection may be accompanied by cutaneous burning sensations and peripheral vasodilation, with moderate fall in BP. Injection should be stopped if patient complains of any discomfort.
- During IV administration, ECG is monitored to detect evidence of hypercalcemia: decreased QT interval associated with inverted T wave.
- Observe IV site closely. Extravasation may result in tissue irritation and necrosis.

CHLORDIAZEPOXIDE

Classes: Sedative-hypnotic; benzodiazepine
Trade Names: APO-chlordiazepoxide (Can), Librium, Novopoxide (Can), Solium (Can).
Therapeutic Action/Pharmacodynamics: Chlordiazepoxide is a benzodiazepine derivative that acts on the limbic,

thalamic, and hypothalamic areas of the CNS. It produces mild sedative, anticonvulsant, and skeletal muscle relaxant effects and has long-acting hypnotic properties.

Emergency Uses: To manage severe anxiety and tension; to manage acute alcohol withdrawal symptoms (delirium tremens). *Adult dose:* 50–100 mg IV/IM.

Pharmacokinetics

Absorption: Slow, erratic absorption if given IM; peak effect is 15–30 min IM, 3–30 min IV; onset is 1–5 min IV; duration is 15–60 min IV.

Distribution: Widely distributed throughout body; crosses the placenta.

Metabolism: Metabolized in liver to long-acting active metabolite.

Elimination: Slowly excreted in urine (may last several days); excreted in breast milk.

Contraindications and Precautions: Contraindicated in hypersensitivity to chlordiazepoxide and other benzodiazepines, pregnancy (category D), nursing mothers, lactation, acute alcohol intoxication, oral use in children under 6 yr, parenteral use in children under 12 yr. Use with caution in patients with primary depressive disorder or psychoses, and acute alcohol intoxication.

Adverse/Side Effects: CNS: Drowsiness, dizziness, lethargy, changes in EEG pattern, vivid dreams, nightmares, headache, vertigo, syncope, tinnitus, confusion, hallucinations, paradoxic rage, depression, delirium, ataxia • CV: Orthostatic hypotension, tachycardia, changes in ECG patterns seen with rapid IV administration • GI: Nausea, dry mouth, vomiting, constipation, increased appetite • GU: Urinary frequency • Other: Edema, pain in injection site, photosensitivity, skin rash, jaundice, hiccups, respiratory depression.

Interactions: It can potentiate CNS depression in patients taking depressants, anticonvulsants, and alcohol. It may increase levels of phenytoin and decrease the antiparkinson effects.

Prehospital Considerations

- Chlordiazepoxide is a Schedule IV controlled substance.
- Prepare parenteral solution immediately before use; discard unused portion. Drug is unstable when exposed to light.
- For IV injection, 5 mL of sterile water for injection or NaCl 0.9% is added to each 100-mg ampule of dry powder and agitated gently until dissolved. Do not use IM diluent for the IV solution because it may contain air bubbles.
- Do not mix any other drug with chlordiazepoxide solution.
- Store in tight, light-resistant containers at 15–30C (59–86F) unless otherwise specified by manufacturer. The special diluent supplied by manufacturer for IM preparation should be kept refrigerated, preferably at 2–8C (36–46F), until ready for use.
- Orthostatic hypotension and tachycardia occur more frequently with parenteral administration. Patient should stay recumbent 2–3 hr after IM or IV injection; observe closely and monitor vital signs.

CHLORPROMAZINE

Classes: Tranquilizer; antipsychotic; phenothiazine
Trade Names: Chlorpromanyl (Can), Largactil (Aus), Novochlorpromazine (Can), Ormazine, Promapar, Promaz, Sonazine, Thorazine, Thor-Prom
Therapeutic Action/Pharmacodynamics: Chlorpromazine is a phenothiazine derivative used to manage severe

psychotic episodes. Phenothiazines are believed to block the postsynaptic dopamine receptors in the brain associated with mood and behavior. Chlorpromazine's actions on the hypothalamus and reticular formation produce strong sedation, hypotension, and depressed temperature regulation. Its inhibitory effect on dopamine reuptake may cause moderate extrapyramidal symptoms. Antipsychotic drugs are sometimes called neuroleptics (or tranquilizers) because they tend to reduce initiative and interest in environment, decrease displays of emotions or affect, suppress spontaneous movements and complex behavior, and decrease psychotic symptoms. They are also used to manage mild alcohol withdrawal, intractable hiccups, and nausea and vomiting.

Emergency Uses: To manage acute psychotic episodes, intractable hiccups, or nausea and vomiting. *Adult dose:* 25–50 mg IM. *Pediatric dose:* 0.5 mg/kg IM; 1.0 mg/kg PR.

Pharmacokinetics
Absorption: Rapid absorption after IM; onset is 30–60 min; peak effect is 15–20 min; duration is 4–6 hr.
Distribution: Widely distributed; accumulates in brain; crosses placenta.
Metabolism: Metabolized in liver.
Elimination: Excreted in urine as metabolites; excreted in breast milk.

Contraindications and Precautions: Chlorpromazine is contraindicated in comatose patients and those who have taken large amounts of sedatives. It is also contraindicated in patients with a hypersensitivity to phenothiazine derivatives; withdrawal states from alcohol; brain damage, bone marrow depression, Reye's syndrome; and in children younger than 6 mo. Safe use during pregnancy (category C) and in nursing mothers is not established. Drug may produce seizures in patients who have taken hallucinogens. It may impair mental and physical abilities and, on occasion, may produce orthostatic hypotension. It has caused extrapyramidal symptoms, especially in children. Use with caution in patients in agitated states accompanied by depression, seizure disorders, or respiratory impairment due to infection or COPD; patients with glaucoma, diabetes, hypertensive disease, peptic ulcer, prostatic hypertrophy, previously detected breast cancer, and those with thyroid, cardiovascular, and hepatic disorders; patients exposed to extreme heat or organophosphate insecticides.

Adverse/Side Effects: Side effects of chlorpromazine are usually dose related. CNS: Sedation, drowsiness, dizziness, restlessness, dyskinesias, tumor, syncope, headache, weakness, insomnia, reduced REM sleep, bizarre dreams, cerebral edema, convulsive seizures, hypothermia, inability to sweat, depressed cough reflex, extrapyramidal symptoms, EEG changes • CV: Orthostatic hypotension, palpitation, tachycardia, ECG changes (usually reversible) including prolonged QT and PR intervals, blunting of T waves, ST depression • Eye: Blurred vision, mydriasis, photophobia • GI: Dry mouth, constipation, ileus, cholestatic jaundice, aggravation of peptic ulcer, dyspepsia, increased appetite • GU: Anovulation, infertility, pseudopregnancy, menstrual irregularity, priapism, inhibition of ejaculation, reduced libido, urinary retention and frequency • Respiratory: Laryngospasm • Skin/hypersensitivity: Urticaria, reduced perspiration, contact dermatitis, exfoliative dermatitis, photosensitivity, eczema, anaphylactoid reactions, hypersensitivity vasculitis; hirsutism (long-term therapy) • Other: Weight gain, hypoglycemia, hyperglycemia, glycosuria (high doses), enlargement of parotid glands, idiopathic edema, muscle necrosis (following IM), sudden unexplained death.

Interactions: Alcohol and other CNS depressants can potentiate CNS depression. Phenobarbital increases the metabolism of chlorpromazine. The antihistamine phenylpropanolamine poses possibility of sudden death; tricyclic antidepressants intensify hypotensive and anticholinergic effects; anticonvulsants decrease seizure threshold (may need to increase anticonvulsant dose to compensate).

Prehospital Considerations

- Avoid parenteral drug contact with skin, eyes, and clothing because of its potential for causing contact dermatitis.
- Inject IM preparations slowly and deep into upper outer quadrant of buttock; massage site well. Avoid SC injection; it may cause tissue irritation and nodule formation. If irritation is a problem, consult physician about diluting medication with normal saline or 2% procaine. Rotate injection sites.
- The patient should remain recumbent for at least 1/2 hr after parenteral administration. Observe closely. Hypotensive reactions may require head-low position and pressor drugs, e.g., phenylephrine (Neo-Synephrine), norepinephrine (Levophed). Epinephrine and other pressor agents are contraindicated since they may cause sudden paradoxical drop in BP.
- Lemon yellow color of parenteral preparation does not alter potency; if otherwise colored or markedly discolored, solution should be discarded.
- Before initiating treatment, establish baseline BP (in standing and recumbent positions), pulse, and respiratory capacity values.
- Hypotensive reactions, dizziness, and sedation are common during early therapy, particularly in patients on high doses and in the elderly receiving parenteral doses. Patients usually develop tolerance to these side effects; however, lower doses or longer intervals between doses may be required.

Chlorpromazine

- Smoking increases metabolism of phenothiazines, resulting in shortened half-life and more rapid clearance of drug. Higher dosage in smokers may be required. Advise patient to stop or at least reduce smoking, if possible.
- Extrapyramidal (EPS) or dystonic reactions are common, especially in children. These should be treated with parenteral diphenhydramine (Benadryl) or benztropine (Cogentin).

DEXAMETHASONE

Class: Steroid

Trade Names: Dalalone, Decadron, Decaject, Dexacen, Dexone, Dexsone, Hexadrol, Solurex

Therapeutic Action/Pharmacodynamics: Dexamethasone is a long-acting synthetic adrenocorticoid with intense anti-inflammatory (glucocorticoid) activity and minimal mineralocorticoid activity. As an anti-inflammatory agent it prevents accumulation of inflammatory cells at sites of infection; inhibits phagocytosis, lysosomal enzyme release, and synthesis of selected chemical mediators of inflammation; reduces capillary dilation and permeability. Dexamethasone is used to manage the inflammatory response seen in allergic reactions. Once thought to significantly decrease cerebral edema, its use in managing brain and spinal cord injury remains controversial. Because a large single dose of steroids has little harmful effect, it is still used frequently in patients with cerebral edema both in the emergency department and in the field.

Emergency Uses: To reduce the inflammatory process in allergic reactions such as anaphylaxis, asthma, and COPD; to reduce cerebral edema. *Adult dose:* 4–24 mg IV/IM. *Pediatric dose:* 0.5–1.0 mg/kg.

Pharmacokinetics

Absorption: Onset and peak effect are less than 1 hr; duration is variable for IV, 6 days IM; half-life is 3.0–4.5 hr. HPA suppression 36–54 hr. (Note: This is more important than the half-life.)

Distribution: Crosses placenta; distributed into breast milk.

Elimination: Hypothalamus-pituitary axis suppression: 36–54 hr.

Contraindications and Precautions: Dexamethasone has no absolute contraindications in the emergency setting. Relative contraindications include patients with systemic fungal infection, acute infections, active or resting tuberculosis, vaccinia, varicella, administration of live virus vaccines (to patient, family members). Use with caution in patients with stromal herpes simplex, keratitis, GI ulceration, renal disease, diabetes mellitus, hypothyroidism, myasthenia gravis, CHF, cirrhosis, psychic disorders, seizures.

Adverse/Side Effects: CNS: Euphoria, insomnia, convulsions, increased ICP, vertigo, headache, psychic disturbances • CV: CHF, hypertension, edema • Endocrine: Menstrual irregularities, hyperglycemia; adrenal insufficiency; growth suppression in children; hirsutism • Eye: Posterior subcapsular cataract, increased IOP, glaucoma, exophthalmos • GI: Peptic ulcer with possible perforation, abdominal distension, nausea, increased appetite, heartburn, dyspepsia, pancreatitis, bowel perforation, oral candidiasis • Musculoskeletal: Muscle weakness, loss of muscle mass, vertebral compression fracture, pathologic fracture of long bones, tendon rupture • Skin: Acne, impaired wound healing, petechiae, ecchymoses, diaphoresis, allergic dermatitis, hypo- or hyperpigmentation, SC and cutaneous atrophy, burning and tingling in perineal area (following IV injection).

Dexamethasone

Interactions: Since barbiturates, phenytoin, and rifampin increase steroid metabolism, the dosage of dexamethasone may need to be increased.

Prehospital Considerations

- Administer IM injection deep into a large muscle mass (e.g., gluteus maximus). Avoid SC injection; atrophy and sterile abscesses may occur.
- The repository form, dexamethasone acetate (for IM or local injection only), is a white suspension that settles on standing; mild shaking will resuspend the drug.
- Dexamethasone may be given undiluted by direct IV over 30 sec or less. Drug may be added to an infusion of D_5W or NS and administered over a prescribed period.
- Cushing's syndrome and other systemic effects can occur. Monitor and report signs and symptoms.

DEXTROSE 50%

Class: Carbohydrate

Trade Names: $D_{50}W$, 50% Dextrose

Therapeutic Action/Pharmacodynamics: Dextrose is the principal form of glucose (sugar) used by the body to create energy. Since serious brain injury can occur in prolonged hypoglycemia, the rapid administration of glucose is essential. Dextrose 50% IV is the treatment of choice for hypoglycemic patients with an altered mental status or no gag reflex.

Emergency Use: To increase blood sugar levels in documented hypoglycemia. *Adult dose:* 25 g of 50% solution IV. *Pediatric dose:* 2 mL/kg of 25% solution IV.

Pharmacokinetics

Absorption: Immediate blood levels; onset <1 min; peak effect and duration dependent upon degree of hypoglycemia.

Distribution: Widely distributed to all body tissues.

Metabolism: Dextrose (glucose) is metabolized to carbon dioxide and water with the release of energy.

Contraindications and Precautions: There are no major contraindications to the IV administration of dextrose 50% to a patient with documented or suspected hypoglycemia. Use with caution in patients with increasing intracranial pressure as the added glucose may worsen the cerebral edema.

Adverse/Side Effects: Patients may complain of warmth, pain, or burning at the injection site. Dextrose 50% can cause tissue necrosis, phlebitis, sclerosis, or thrombosis at the injection site. Dextrose can cause severe neurologic symptoms (Wernicke's encephalopathy, Korsakoff's psychosis) if patient is thiamine deficient. Use with 100 mg thiamine in patients suspected of having thiamine deficiency.

Interactions: None in the emergency setting.

Prehospital Considerations

- Always ensure a patent IV line before administering dextrose 50% as severe tissue necrosis may occur with extravasation of this solution.
- Report and record blood glucose levels before and after administering this solution.

DIAZEPAM

Classes: Sedative-hypnotic; anticonvulsant; benzodiazepine; antianxiety

Trade Names: Apodiazepam (Can), Atenex (Aus), Diazemuls (Can, Aus), Ducene (Aus), Novo-Dipam (Can), Valium, Zetran

Therapeutic Action/Pharmacodynamics: Diazepam is a benzodiazepine whose exact mechanism is unknown, but many believe it appears to act at both limbic and subcortical levels of the CNS. It is principally used for its anticonvulsant properties; it suppresses the spread of seizure activity through motor cortex of the brain. It does not appear to abolish the abnormal electrical discharge focus. It is also used as a sedative in the management of stress and anxiety and to treat the withdrawal symptoms of alcohol. Diazepam is an effective skeletal muscle relaxant, making it an effective adjunct in managing orthopedic injuries. It is also useful as a premedication for minor surgeries and cardioversion because it induces amnesia, which diminishes the patient's recall of the procedure.

Emergency Uses: To stop seizure activity, especially status epilepticus. *Adult dose:* 5–10 mg IV/IM. *Pediatric dose:* 0.5–2 mg IV/IM.

To manage acute anxiety. *Adult dose:* 2–5 mg IM. *Pediatric dose:* 0.5–2 mg IM.

As premedication for cardioversion. *Adult dose:* 5–15 mg IV. *Pediatric dose:* 0.2–0.5 mg/kg IV.

Pharmacokinetics
Absorption: Erratic IM absorption; onset is 1–5 min IV, 15–30 min IM; peak effect in 15 min IV, 30–45 min IM; duration is 15–60 min; half-life is 20–50 hr.
Distribution: Crosses blood-brain barrier and placenta; distributed into breast milk.
Metabolism: Metabolized in liver to active metabolites.
Elimination: Excreted primarily in urine.

Contraindications and Precautions: Diazepam is contraindicated in patients with a hypersensitivity to the drug. IV diazepam is contraindicated in shock, coma, acute alcohol intoxication, depressed vital signs, obstetrical patients, infants less than 30 days old. Use with caution in patients with psychoses, mental depression;

myasthenia gravis; impaired hepatic or renal function; and in individuals who are known to abuse drugs or be addiction-prone. Use IV diazepam with extreme caution in the elderly, the very ill, and patients with COPD.

Adverse/Side Effects: CNS: Drowsiness, fatigue, ataxia, confusion, paradoxic rage, dizziness, vertigo, amnesia, vivid dreams, headache, slurred speech, tremor; EEG changes, tardive dyskinesia • CV: Hypotension, tachycardia, edema, cardiovascular collapse • Eye: Blurred vision, diplopia, nystagmus • GI: Nausea, constipation • GU: Incontinence, urinary retention, gynecomastia (prolonged use), menstrual irregularities • Other: Hiccups, coughing, throat and chest pain, laryngospasm, ovulation failure, pain, venous thrombosis, phlebitis at injection site, hepatic dysfunction.

Interactions: Alcohol, CNS depressants, and anticonvulsants can potentiate CNS depression. Cimetidine increases diazepam plasma levels and toxicity. Diazepam may decrease the antiparkinson effects of levodopa and increase phenytoin levels. Smoking decreases its sedative and antianxiety effects.

Prehospital Considerations
- IM administration should be made deep into large muscle mass. Inject slowly. Alternate injection sites.
- To prevent swelling, irritation, venous thrombosis, and phlebitis, give direct IV by injecting drug slowly, taking at least 1 min for each 5 mg (1 mL) given to adults and taking at least 3 min to inject 0.25 mg/kg body weight of children.
- Avoid small veins; extreme care should be taken to avoid intra-arterial administration or extravasation.
- Because diazepam is a relatively short-acting drug, seizure activity may recur and additional doses may be required.

- Preserve in tight, light-resistant containers at 15–30C (59–86F), unless otherwise specified by manufacturer.
- When diazepam is given parenterally, hypotension, muscular weakness, tachycardia, and respiratory depression may occur. Observe patient closely and monitor vital signs.
- Smoking increases metabolism of diazepam; therefore, clinical effectiveness is lowered. Heavy smokers may need a higher dose than nonsmokers.
- Flumazenil (Romazicon) is an effective benzodiazepine antagonist and should be available in case respiratory depression or other complications ensue.

DIAZOXIDE

Class: Antihypertensive

Trade Name: Hyperstat

Therapeutic Action/Pharmacodynamics: Rapid-acting thiazide (benzothiadiazine) nondiuretic hypotensive and hyperglycemic agent. In contrast to thiazide diuretics, causes sodium and water retention and decreases urinary output, probably because it increases proximal tubular reabsorption of sodium and decreases glomerular filtration rate. Reduces peripheral vascular resistance and BP by direct vasodilatory effect on peripheral arteriolar smooth muscles, perhaps by direct competition for calcium receptor sites. Its hypotensive effect may be accompanied by marked reflex increase in heart rate, cardiac output, and stroke volume; thus cerebral and coronary blood flow are usually maintained.

Emergency Use: To rapidly decrease BP in hypertensive crisis. *Adult dose:* 1–3 mg/kg IV up to 150 mg given over 30 sec repeated at 5–15 min intervals as needed. *Pediatric dose:* Same as adult.

Diazoxide

Pharmacokinetics

Absorption: Onset in 30–60 sec IV; peak effect in 5 min; duration is 2–12 hr or more; half-life is 21–45 hr.
Distribution: Crosses blood-brain barrier and placenta.
Metabolism: Partially metabolized in the liver.
Elimination: Excreted in urine.

Contraindications and Precautions: Patients with a hypersensitivity to diazoxide or to other thiazides, cerebral bleeding, eclampsia, and significant coronary artery disease. Safe use during pregnancy (category C) and in nursing mothers is not established. Use with caution in patients with diabetes mellitus, impaired cerebral or cardiac circulation, or impaired renal function; in patients taking corticosteroids or estrogen-progesterone combinations; and in those with a history of gout or uremia.

Adverse/Side Effects: CNS: Tinnitus, momentary hearing loss, headache, weakness, malaise, dizziness, sleepiness, insomnia, euphoria, anxiety, extrapyramidal signs • CV: Palpitations, atrial and ventricular dysrhythmias, flushing, shock; orthostatic hypotension, CHF, transient hypertension • Eye: Blurred vision, transient cataracts, subconjunctival hemorrhage, diplopia, lacrimation, papilledema • GI: Nausea, vomiting, abdominal discomfort, diarrhea, constipation, ileus, anorexia, transient loss of taste • Hypersensitivity: Rash, fever • Renal: Decreased urinary output, nephrotic syndrome (reversible), hematuria, increased nocturia, proteinuria, azotemia • Skin: Pruritus, flushing, monilial dermatitis, herpes, hirsutism; loss of scalp hair, sweating, sensation of warmth, burning, or itching. Other: hyperglycemia, edema, sodium and water retention.

Interactions: The effects of diazoxide can be potentiated when it is administered with other antihypertensive agents. It can also increase phenytoin metabolism, decreasing the blood levels of phenytoin and precipitating seizures.

Prehospital Considerations

- Hypotension may occur and, if severe, should be treated with sympathomimetics. Because of the rapid onset of diazoxide, frequent monitoring of vital signs is essential to detect a drop in peripheral perfusion. Tachycardia has occurred immediately following IV administration; palpitations and bradycardia have also been reported.
- Since diazoxide causes sodium and water retention, a diuretic is generally prescribed to avoid CHF and drug resistance and to maximize hypotensive effect.
- When a diuretic, e.g., furosemide (Lasix), is prescribed, it is generally given 30–60 min prior to IV diazoxide. Patient should remain recumbent 8–10 hr because of possible additive hypotensive effect.
- Check the IV injection site frequently. The solution is strongly alkaline. Extravasation of medication into SC or IV tissues can cause severe inflammatory reaction. Diazoxide is administered only by peripheral vein.
- If BP continues to fall 30 min or more after IV drug administration, suspect cause other than drug effect. Notify physician immediately.

DIGOXIN

Class: Cardiac glycoside
Trade Names: Digoxin, Lanoxin, Novodigoxin (Can)
Therapeutic Action/Pharmacodynamics: Digoxin is a rapid-acting cardiac glycoside used in the treatment of congestive heart failure and rapid atrial dysrhythmias. It acts by increasing the force and velocity of myocardial systolic contraction through its effects on the sodium-potassium ATPase system. By significantly increasing stroke volume,

it increases cardiac output (positive inotropic effect). It also decreases conduction velocity through the atrioventricular node. Action is more prompt and less prolonged than that of digitalis and digitoxin, thus decreasing the heart rate (negative chronotropic and dromotropic effects). It is less likely than digitoxin or digitalis to give rise to cumulative effects because it is more readily absorbed and exchanged in the body and is rather rapidly excreted in urine.

Emergency Uses: To increase cardiac output in congestive heart failure and to stabilize supraventricular tachydys-rhythmias, especially atrial flutter and atrial fibrillation. *Adult dose:* 0.25–0.5 mg slow IV. *Pediatric dose:* 10–50 mcg/kg (age dependent) IV.

Pharmacokinetics
Absorption: Onset is 5–30 min; peak effect is 1–5 hr; duration is 3–4 days in fully digitalized patient; half-life is 34–44 hr.
Distribution: Widely distributed; tissue levels significantly higher than plasma levels; crosses placenta.
Metabolism: Approximately 14% in liver.
Elimination: 80–90% excreted by kidneys; may appear in breast milk.

Contraindications and Precautions: Digoxin is contraindicated in digitalis hypersensitivity, ventricular fibrillation, ventricular tachycardia unless due to CHF. Full digitalizing dose not given if patient has received digoxin during previous week or if slowly excreted cardiotonic glycoside has been given during previous 2 wk. Use with extreme caution in patients with acute MI as they are prone to digoxin toxicity. Digoxin toxicity is potentiated in patients with hypokalemia, hypocalcemia, hypomagnesemia, advanced heart disease, incomplete AV block, cor pulmonale, hyperthyroidism, lung disease, pregnancy (category A), nursing women, premature and immature infants, children, and elderly or debilitated patients. Since it crosses the placenta, it can affect fetal heart tones in the same manner as the mother's.

Adverse/Side Effects: CNS: Fatigue, muscle weakness, headache, facial neuralgia, mental depression, paresthesias, hallucinations, confusion, drowsiness, agitation, dizziness • CV: Dysrhythmias, hypotension, AV block • Eye: Visual disturbances • GI: Anorexia, nausea, vomiting, diarrhea • Other: Diaphoresis, recurrent malaise, dysphagia.

Interactions: Quinidine, amiodarone, and calcium channel blockers (verapamil, nifedipine, diltiazem) can increase serum digoxin levels. Severe bradycardia can occur if digoxin is administered with IV beta blockers. Diuretics can cause potassium depletion, which can lead to digoxin toxicity. Succinylcholine may potentiate the dysrhythmogenic effects of digoxin.

Prehospital Considerations

- IV administration: Direct IV injection of digoxin may be administered undiluted or diluted in 4 mL of sterile water, D_5W, or NaCl 0.9% (if prescribed). Administer each direct IV dose over at least 5 min.
- Infiltration of parenteral drug into subcutaneous tissue can cause local irritation and sloughing.
- Be familiar with patient's baseline data (e.g., quality of peripheral pulses, blood pressure, clinical symptoms, serum electrolytes, creatinine clearance) as a foundation for making assessments.
- Before administering digoxin, check laboratory reports for serum levels of digoxin, potassium, magnesium, and calcium. Notify physician of abnormal changes.
- Before administering digoxin, take apical pulse for 1 full min, noting rate, rhythm, and quality. If changes are

Digoxin

noted, withhold digoxin, take rhythm strip if patient is on ECG monitor, and notify physician promptly.

- Monitor for signs and symptoms of digoxin toxicity.
- Although a fall in ventricular rate to 60/min in adults (70/min in children) is one criterion for withholding medication, any change in pulse rate or rhythm should be interpreted as a sign of digitalis intoxication and should be reported promptly.
- In children, cardiac dysrhythmias are usually reliable signs of early toxicity. Early indicators in adults (anorexia, nausea, vomiting, diarrhea, visual disturbances) are rarely initial signs in children.

DIGOXIN IMMUNE FAB

Class: Antidote

Trade Name: Digibind

Therapeutic Action/Pharmacodynamics: Digoxin Immune Fab consists of purified fragments of antibodies specific for digoxin (but also effective for digitoxin) produced in sheep immunized with digoxin-albumin conjugate. Using fragments of antidigoxin antibodies (Fab) instead of whole antibody molecules permits more extensive and faster distribution to serum and toxic cellular sites. It acts by selectively forming a complex with circulating digoxin or digitoxin, thereby preventing the drug from binding at receptor sites; the complex is then eliminated in urine.

Emergency Uses: To treat potentially life-threatening digoxin or digitoxin intoxication in carefully selected patients. *Adult dose:* Dosages vary according to amount of digoxin to be neutralized; dosages are based on total body load or steady state serum digoxin concentrations (see package insert); some patients may require a second dose after several hours.

Pharmacokinetics

Absorption: Onset is within 1 min after IV administration; half-life is 14–20 hr.

Elimination: Excreted in urine over 5–7 days.

Contraindications and Precautions: Digoxin Immune Fab is contraindicated in patients with a hypersensitivity to sheep products; renal or cardiac failure. Safe use during pregnancy (category C) or in nursing mothers is not established. Use with caution in patients with prior treatment with sheep antibodies or ovine Fab fragments; history of allergies; impaired renal function.

Adverse/Side Effects: Adverse reactions associated with use of Digoxin Immune Fab are related primarily to the effects of digitalis withdrawal on the heart. Allergic reactions have been reported rarely. Hypokalemia.

Interactions: None established.

Prehospital Considerations

- Reconstitute by dissolving 38 mg (1 vial) in 4 mL of sterile water for injection; mix gently (solution will contain 9.5 mg/mL). For administration by IV infusion, reconstituted solution may be diluted further with sterile isotonic saline injection.
- After reconstitution, Digoxin Immune Fab is administered by IV infusion over 30 min, preferably through a 0.22-mm membrane filter, or as a bolus injection if cardiac arrest is imminent.
- For infants, reconstitute as directed and administer with a tuberculin syringe. For small doses (e.g., 2 mg or less), dilute the reconstituted 40-mg vial with 40 mL of sterile isotonic saline injection to make a concentration of 1 mg/mL. Children must be closely monitored for fluid overload.
- Reconstituted solutions should be used promptly or refrigerated at 2–8C (36–46F) for up to 4 hr.

- Effective treatment should be reflected in improvement in cardiac rhythm abnormalities, mental orientation, and other neurologic symptoms, and GI and visual disturbances.
- Reversal of signs and symptoms of digitalis toxicity occurs in 15–60 min in adults and usually within minutes in children.
- Cardiac status may deteriorate as inotropic action of digitalis is withdrawn by action of Digoxin Immune Fab. Closely monitor for CHF, dysrhythmias, increase in heart rate, and hypokalemia.

DILTIAZEM

Class: Calcium channel blocker

Trade Names: Apo-Diltiaz (Can), Cardizem, Dilacor, Tiazac

Therapeutic Actions/Pharmacodynamics: Diltiazem is a slow calcium channel blocker with pharmacologic actions similar to those of verapamil. It inhibits calcium ion influx through slow channels into cells of myocardial and arterial smooth muscle (both coronary and peripheral blood vessels). As a result, intracellular calcium remains at subthreshold levels insufficient to stimulate cell excitation and contraction. It also dilates coronary arteries and arterioles and inhibits coronary artery spasm; thus myocardial oxygen delivery is increased (antianginal effect). Diltiazem slows SA and AV node conduction (antidysrhythmic effect) without affecting normal atrial action potential or intraventricular conduction. By vasodilation of peripheral arterioles it decreases total peripheral vascular resistance and reduces arterial BP at rest (antihypertensive effect). It may cause slight decrease in heart rate without altering total serum calcium levels.

Emergency Uses: To control supraventricular tachydys-rhythmias (atrial fibrillation, atrial flutter, PSVT refractory to adenosine); to increase coronary artery perfusion in angina pectoris. *Adult dose:* 0.25 mg/kg IV bolus over 2 min; if inadequate response, may repeat in 15 min with 0.35 mg/kg, followed by a continuous infusion of 5–10 mg/hr (recommended maximum dose: 15 mg/hr for 24 hr).

Pharmacokinetics
Absorption: Onset is 3 min; peak effect in 7 min; duration is 1–3 hr; half-life is 2 hr.
Distribution: Distributed into breast milk.
Metabolism: Metabolized in liver.
Elimination: Excreted primarily in urine with some elimination in feces.

Contraindications and Precautions: Diltiazem is contraindicated in patients with a known hypersensitivity to the drug; sick sinus syndrome (unless pacemaker is in place and functioning); second- or third-degree AV block; severe hypotension (systolic less than 90 mm Hg or diastolic less than 60 mm Hg). Do not use in patients with wide-complex tachycardia (ventricular tachycardia) in the prehospital setting. Do not use if patient has Wolf-Parkinson-White syndrome. Its safe use in pregnancy (category C), in nursing mothers, and in children has not been established. Use with caution in CHF (especially if patient is also receiving a beta blocker), conduction abnormalities; renal or hepatic impairment; the elderly; nursing mothers.

Adverse/Side Effects: CNS: Headache, fatigue, dizziness, asthenia, drowsiness, nervousness, insomnia, confusion, tremor, gait abnormality • CV: Edema, dysrhythmias, angina, second- or third-degree AV block, bradycardia, CHF, flushing, hypotension, syncope, palpitations • GI: Nausea, constipation, anorexia, vomiting, diarrhea, impaired taste, weight increase • Skin: Rash.

Interactions: Digoxin should not be used with IV calcium channel blockers because of the increased risk of congestive heart failure, bradycardia, and asystole. Diltiazem may increase digoxin or quinidine levels. Cimetidine may increase diltiazem levels, thus increasing its effects. Diltiazem may increase cyclosporine levels.

Prehospital Considerations

- Calcium chloride can be used to prevent the hypotensive effects of diltiazem in overdose situations.
- Diltiazem may be given by direct IV as a bolus dose over 2 min. A second bolus may be administered after 15 min.
- Diltiazem may be given by continuous IV infusion. The recommended rate is 5–15 mg/hr. Infusion duration longer than 24 hr and infusion rate greater than 15 mg/hr are not recommended.
- For continuous IV infusion, diltiazem may be added to any of the following: D_5W, NS, D_5W/0.45% NaCl.
- Diltiazem should be kept refrigerated but can be kept at room temperature for 1 month, then discarded if not used.
- Withhold drug if systolic BP is less than 90 mm Hg or diastolic is less than 60 mm Hg.
- BP and ECG should be evaluated before initiation of therapy and monitored particularly during dosage adjustment period.

DIMENHYDRINATE

Class: Antihistamine

Trade Names: Andrumin (Aus), Apo-Dimenhydrinate (Can), Dinate, Dommanate, Dramamine, Gravol (Can), Marmine, Nauseatol (Can), Novo-Dimanate (Can), Travamine (Can)

Therapeutic Action/Pharmacodynamics: Dimenhydrinate is an H_1-receptor antagonist that shares similar properties with diphenhydramine. Although formally classified as an antihistamine, it is rarely used for this purpose. It is most often used in the prevention and treatment of motion sickness, vertigo, and labrynthitis. Its precise mode of antinauseant action is not known, but it is thought to inhibit cholinergic stimulation in vestibular and associated neural pathways. It also is used with analgesics, particularly narcotics.

Emergency Uses: To relieve nausea/vomiting associated with motion sickness and narcotic use. *Adult dose:* 12.5–25 mg IV; 50 mg IM every 4 hr as needed. *Pediatric dose:* 1.25 mg/kg every 4 hr up to 300 mg/day.

Pharmacokinetics
Absorption: Onset is immediate if given IV; 20–30 min IM; duration is 3–6 hr.
Distribution: Distributed into breast milk.
Elimination: Excreted in urine.

Contraindications and Precautions: There are no absolute contraindications when used in the emergency setting. Use with caution in patients with seizure disorders and asthma.

Adverse/Side Effects: CNS: Drowsiness, headache, incoordination, dizziness, blurred vision, nervousness, restlessness, insomnia (especially in children) • CV: Hypotension, palpitation • Other: Dry mouth, nose, throat • Less frequently: Anorexia, constipation, or diarrhea, urinary frequency, dysuria.

Interactions: Alcohol and other CNS depressants enhance CNS depression, drowsiness. Tricyclic antidepressants compound its anticholinergic effects.

Prehospital Considerations
- Dimenhydrinate may be given by direct IV. Dilute each 50 mg in 10 mL of NS. Administer 50 mg or fraction thereof over 2 min.

- Examine parenteral preparation for particulate matter and discoloration. Do not use unless absolutely clear.
- Causes high incidence of drowsiness. Side rails and supervision of ambulation may be indicated.
- Tolerance to CNS depressant effects usually occurs after a few days of drug therapy. Some decrease in antiemetic action may result with prolonged use.
- Antihistamines can obscure signs of dizziness, nausea, and vomiting associated with drug toxicity and serious disease conditions.
- To prevent motion sickness, dimenhydrinate should be taken 30 min before departure and should be repeated before meals and upon retiring.

DIMERCAPROL

Class: Antidote

Trade Name: BAL in Oil

Therapeutic Action/Pharmacodynamics: Dimercaprol is a dithiol compound that combines with ions of various heavy metals to form relatively stable, nontoxic, soluble complexes called chelates, which can be excreted. This action prevents the inhibition of sulfhydryl enzymes by toxic metal. It may also reactivate affected enzymes but is most effective when administered prior to enzyme damage.

Emergency Uses: As an antidote for acute arsenic and gold poisoning. *Adult dose:* 2.5–3.0 mg/kg IM. *Pediatric dose:* Same as for adult.

As an antidote for acute mercury poisoning. *Adult dose:* 5 mg/kg IM. *Pediatric dose:* Same as for adult.

As an antidote for acute lead encephalopathy. *Adult dose:* 4 mg/kg IM. *Pediatric dose:* Same as for adult.

Pharmacokinetics

Absorption: Onset and peak effect in 30–60 min.
Distribution: Distributed mainly in intracellular spaces, including brain; highest concentrations in liver and kidneys.
Elimination: Completely excreted in urine and bile within 4 hr.

Contraindications and Precautions: Dimercaprol is contraindicated in hepatic insufficiency (with exception of postarsenical jaundice); severe renal insufficiency; poisoning due to cadmium, iron, selenium, or uranium. Use with caution in hypertensive patients. Safe use during pregnancy (category D) and in nursing mothers not established.

Adverse/Side Effects: CNS: Headache, anxiety, muscle pain or weakness, restlessness, paresthesias, tremors, convulsions, shock • CV: Elevated BP, tachycardia • ENT: Rhinorrhea; burning sensation, feeling of pain and constriction in throat • GI: Nausea, vomiting; burning sensation in lips and mouth, halitosis, salivation; abdominal pain, metabolic acidosis • GU: Burning sensation in penis, renal damage • Other: Pains in chest or hands, pain and sterile abscess at injection site, sweating, dental pain.

Interactions: Iron, cadmium, selenium, and uranium form toxic complexes with dimercaprol.

Prehospital Considerations

- Because irreversible tissue damage may occur quickly, particularly in mercury poisoning, dimercaprol therapy must be initiated as soon as possible (within 1–2 hr) after ingestion of the poison.
- Administered by deep IM injection only. Local pain, gluteal abscess, and skin sensitization have been reported.
- Contact of drug with skin may produce erythema, edema, dermatitis. Handle with caution.

- Presence of sediment in ampule reportedly does not indicate drug deterioration.
- Monitor vital signs. Elevations of systolic and diastolic BPs accompanied by tachycardia frequently occur within a few minutes following injection and may remain elevated up to 2 hr.
- Fever occurs in approximately 30% of children receiving treatment and may persist throughout therapy.
- Minor adverse reactions usually reach maximum levels 15–20 min after drug administration and generally subside in 30–90 min. Ephedrine or an antihistamine is sometimes administered to prevent symptoms.

DIPHENHYDRAMINE

Class: Antihistamine

Trade Name: Benadryl

Therapeutic Action/Pharmacodynamics:
Diphenhydramine is an antihistamine with significant anticholinergic activity. It is useful for treating allergic reaction and anaphylaxis. High incidence of drowsiness, but GI side effects are minor. Diphenhydramine competes for H_1-receptor sites on effector cells, thus blocking histamine release. Its effects in parkinsonism and drug-induced extrapyramidal symptoms are apparently related to its ability to suppress central cholinergic activity and to prolong action of dopamine by inhibiting its reuptake and storage. It does not inhibit gastric secretion but has strong antiemetic effect.

Emergency Uses: To decrease the effects of allergic reactions and the extrapyramidal symptoms following an antipsychotic medication. *Adult dose:* 25–50 mg IV/IM. *Pediatric dose:* 2–5 mg/kg IV/IM.

Pharmacokinetics

Absorption: Onset is 15–30 min; duration is under 10 min.
Distribution: Widely distributed; does not cross blood-brain barrier.
Metabolism: Inactive in the liver, kidney, and plasma by monoamine oxidase and COMT.
Elimination: Excreted in urine.

Contraindications and Precautions: Contraindicated in hypersensitivity to antihistamines of similar structure; lower respiratory tract symptoms (including acute asthma); narrow-angle glaucoma; prostatic hypertrophy, bladder neck obstruction; GI obstruction or stenosis; pregnancy (category C), nursing mothers, premature infants, and newborns; use as nighttime sleep aid in children under age 12. Use with caution in patients with a history of asthma; convulsive disorders; increased intraocular pressure; hyperthyroidism; hypertension, cardiovascular disease; diabetes mellitus; elderly patients, infants, and young children.

Adverse/Side Effects: CNS: Drowsiness, dizziness, headache, fatigue, disturbed coordination, tingling, heaviness and weakness of hands, tremors, euphoria, nervousness, restlessness, insomnia, confusion (especially in children), excitement, fever • CV: Palpitation, tachycardia, mild hypotension or hypertension, cardiovascular collapse • ENT: Tinnitus, vertigo, dry nose, throat, nasal stuffiness • Eye: Blurred vision, diplopia, photosensitivity, dry eyes • GI: Dry mouth, nausea, epigastric distress, anorexia, vomiting, constipation, or diarrhea • GU: Urinary frequency or retention, dysuria • Hypersensitivity: Skin rash, urticaria, photosensitivity, anaphylactic shock • Respiratory: Thickened bronchial secretions, wheezing, sensation of chest tightness.

Interactions: Alcohol and other CNS depressants, MAO inhibitors compound CNS depression.

Prehospital Considerations

- Administer IM injection deep into large muscle mass; alternate injection sites. Avoid perivascular or SC injections of the drug because of its irritating effects. Hypersensitivity reactions (including anaphylactic shock) are more likely to occur with parenteral injections than with PO administration.
- IV diphenhydramine may be given by direct IV undiluted at a rate of 25 mg or a fraction thereof over 1 min.
- Patients with blood pressure problems who are receiving the drug parenterally should be closely monitored.

DOBUTAMINE

Class: Sympathomimetic

Trade Name: Dobutrex

Therapeutic Action/Pharmacodynamics: Dobutamine produces its inotropic effect by acting on beta receptors and primarily on myocardial alpha-adrenergic receptors. It increases cardiac output (positive inotropic effect) and decreases pulmonary wedge pressure and total systemic vascular resistance with comparatively little or no effect on BP or heart rate. Its primary use is inotropic support in short-term treatment of adults with cardiac decompensation due to depressed myocardial contractility (cardiogenic shock) resulting from either organic heart disease or cardiac surgery. Dobutamine also increases conduction through the AV node. It has lower potential for precipitating dysrhythmias than dopamine. In CHF, increasing cardiac output enhances renal perfusion and increases renal output and renal sodium excretion.

Emergency Uses: To increase cardiac output in congestive heart failure/cardiogenic shock. *Adult dose:* 2–20 mcg/kg/min IV. *Pediatric dose:* Same as adult.

Pharmacokinetics
Absorption: Onset is 2–10 min; peak effect in 10–20 min; half-life is 2 min.
Metabolism: Metabolized in liver and other tissues by catechol-o-methyl-transferase (COMT).
Elimination: Excreted in urine.

Contraindications and Precautions: Dobutamine is contraindicated in patients with a history of hypersensitivity to other sympathomimetic amines, ventricular tachycardia, or idiopathic hypertrophic subaortic stenosis. Safe use in pregnancy (category C), in nursing mothers, and in children, or following acute MI is not established. Use with caution in patients with preexisting hypertension or atrial fibrillation. Dobutamine should not be used as a sole agent in managing hypovolemic shock until fluid volume is restored. To increase cardiac output in severe emergencies, such as cardiogenic shock, dopamine is the drug of choice.

Adverse/Side Effects: CNS: Headache, tremors, paresthesias, mild leg cramps, nervousness, fatigue (with overdosage) • CV: Increased heart rate and BP, premature ventricular beats, palpitation, anginal pain • GI: Nausea, vomiting • Other: Nonspecific chest pain, shortness of breath.

Interactions: Beta-adrenergic blocking agents, e.g., metoprolol or propranolol, may make dobutamine ineffective in increasing cardiac output, but total peripheral resistance may increase. Since MAO inhibitors and tricylic antidepressants may potentiate the vasopressor effects of dobutamine, use with extreme caution.

Prehospital Considerations
• Hypovolemia should be corrected by administration of appropriate volume expanders prior to initiation of therapy.

- Since dobutamine enhances AV conduction, patients with atrial fibrillation are generally given a digitalis preparation prior to initiation of therapy to reduce risk of ventricular tachycardia.
- Rate of infusion should be controlled by an infusion pump (preferred) or a microdrip IV infusion set.
- Solutions containing dobutamine may exhibit color changes because of slight oxidation of drug. This does not affect potency.
- Dobutamine is incompatible with sodium bicarbonate and other alkaline solutions.
- At any given dosage level, drug takes 10–20 min to produce peak effects.
- ECG and BP should be monitored continuously during administration of dobutamine.
- IV infusion rate and duration of therapy are determined by heart rate, blood pressure, and ectopic activity.
- Marked increases in blood pressure (systolic pressure is the most likely to be affected) and heart rate, or the appearance of dysrhythmias or other adverse cardiac effects, are usually reversed promptly by reduction in dosage.
- Patients with preexisting hypertension must be closely observed for exaggerated pressor response.

DOPAMINE

Class: Sympathomimetic

Trade Names: Intropin, Revimine (Can)

Therapeutic Action/Pharmacodynamics: Dopamine is a naturally occurring neurotransmitter and immediate precursor of norepinephrine. Its major cardiovascular effects are produced by direct action on alpha- and beta-adrenergic receptors and on specific dopaminergic receptors in mesenteric and renal vascular beds. Its positive inotropic effect on myocardium increases cardiac output with increase in systolic and pulse pressure and little or no effect on diastolic pressure. Dopamine improves circulation to the renal vascular bed by decreasing renal vascular resistance with a resulting increase in glomerular filtration rate and urinary output.

Emergency Uses: To increase end-organ perfusion in cardiogenic shock and in hemodynamically significant hypotension (70–100 mmHg) not resulting from hypovolemia. *Adult dose:* 2–5 mcg/kg/min up to 20 mcg/kg/min, titrated to effect. *Pediatric dose:* Same as adult.

Pharmacokinetics
Absorption: Onset is less than 5 min; duration is less than 10 min; half-life is 2 min.
Distribution: Widely distributed; does not cross blood-brain barrier.
Metabolism: Inactivated in the liver, kidney, and plasma by MAO and COMT.
Elimination: Excreted in urine.

Contraindications and Precautions: Dopamine is contraindicated in patients with pheochromocytoma (adrenal gland tumor), tachydysrhythmias, or ventricular fibrillation. Safe use during pregnancy (category C), in nursing women, and in children is not established. Cautious use in patients with history of occlusive vascular disease (e.g., Buerger's or Raynaud's disease), cold injury, diabetic endarteritis, or arterial embolism. Always ensure patient is normovolemic prior to using dopamine for hypovolemic shock. Infusion rates above 20 mcg/kg/min will cause profound vasoconstriction because of the drug's predominantly alpha stimulation at that dose range.

Adverse/Side Effects: CV: Hypotension, ectopic beats, tachycardia, anginal pain, palpitation, vasoconstriction (indicated by disproportionate rise in diastolic pressure), cold extremities; less frequent: aberrant conduction, bradycardia, widening of QRS complex, elevated blood pressure • GI: Nausea, vomiting • Other: Headache, necrosis, tissue sloughing with extravasation, gangrene, azotemia, piloerection, dyspnea, dilated pupils (high doses).

Interactions: Like all catecholamines, dopamine is deactivated by alkaline solutions such as sodium bicarbonate. MAO inhibitors increase the alpha-adrenergic effects of dopamine and cause headache, hyperpyrexia, and hypertension. Phenytoin may decrease dopamine action and actually cause hypotensive effects. Beta blockers will antagonize its cardiac effects just as alpha blockers will antagonize peripheral vasoconstriction.

Prehospital Considerations

- Before initiation of dopamine therapy, hypovolemia should be corrected.
- IV infusion rate and guidelines for adjusting rate of flow are in relation to changes in blood pressure. Microdrip or another reliable metering device should be used for accuracy of flow rate.
- Infusion rate must be continuously monitored for free flow, and care must be taken to avoid extravasation, which can result in tissue sloughing and gangrene. For this reason, infusion is made preferably into a large vein of the antecubital fossa.
- Protect dopamine from light. Discolored solutions should not be used.
- Monitor blood pressure, pulse, and peripheral pulses every 5 min. Precise measurements are essential for accurate titration of dosage.
- Close observation is critical when patient is receiving dopamine. The following indicators are used for

decreasing or temporarily suspending dose (report promptly to physician): ascending tachycardia; dysrhythmias; disproportionate rise in diastolic pressure (marked decrease in pulse pressure); signs of peripheral ischemia (pallor, cyanosis, mottling, coldness, complaints of tenderness, pain, numbness, or burning sensation). Presence of peripheral pulses is not always indicative of adequate circulation.

- In addition to improvement in vital signs, other indices of adequate dosage and perfusion of vital organs include loss of pallor, increase in toe temperature, adequacy of nail bed capillary filling, and reversal of confusion or comatose state.

DROPERIDOL

Class: Antiemetic

Trade Name: Inapsine

Therapeutic Action/Pharmacodynamics: Droperidol is a butyrophenone derivative structurally and pharmacologically related to haloperidol. It antagonizes emetic effects of morphine-like analgesics and other drugs that act on the chemoreceptor trigger zone (CTZ). Its mild alpha-adrenergic blocking activity and direct vasodilator effect may cause hypotension. Droperidol acts primarily at the subcortical level to produce sedation. Its sedative property reduces anxiety and motor activity without necessarily inducing sleep, so the patient remains responsive. It potentiates other CNS depressants.

Emergency Uses: To reduce nausea and vomiting in patients refractory to the first-line antiemetics (promethazine, chlorpromazine, etc.) and to produce a tranquilizing effect. It also can be used as an antipsychotic in patients showing marked psychosis requiring

pharmacologic therapy. *Adult dose:* 2.5–10.0 mg IV.
Pediatric dose: 0.088–0.165 mg/kg IV.

Pharmacokinetics

Absorption: Onset is 3–10 min; peak effect in 30 min; duration is 2–4 hr; may persist up to 12 hr.
Distribution: Crosses placenta.
Metabolism: Metabolized in liver.
Elimination: Excreted in urine and feces.

Contraindications and Precautions: Droperidol is contraindicated in patients with a known intolerance to the drug. Safe use during pregnancy (category C) and in children under 2 yr is not established. Use with caution in elderly, debilitated, and other poor-risk patients; and in patients with Parkinson's disease, hypotension, liver, kidney, or cardiac disease, bradydysrhythmias. Droperidol has received an FDA "black box" warning because of prolonging the QTc interval and possible dysrhythmogenesis.

Adverse/Side Effects: CNS: Drowsiness, extrapyramidal symptoms: dystonia, akathisia, oculogyric crisis; dizziness, restlessness, anxiety, hallucinations, mental depression • CV: Hypotension, tachycardia • Other: Chills, shivering, laryngospasm, bronchospasm.

Interactions: None reported.

Prehospital Considerations

- When patient is under the effect of another CNS depressant, the required dose of droperidol may be less than usual. Postoperative narcotics or other CNS depressants are prescribed in reduced doses since they have additive or potentiating effects.
- Protect from light. Store at 15–30C (59–86F), unless otherwise directed by manufacturer.
- Monitor vital signs closely. Hypotension and tachycardia are common side effects. If possible, obtain a 12-lead ECG before administration.

Droperidol

- Because of possibility of severe orthostatic hypotension, always exercise care in moving and positioning the medicated patient. Avoid abrupt changes in position.
- Patient who receives a narcotic analgesic concurrently should be observed carefully for signs of impending respiratory depression.
- Elevated BP has been reported following administration of droperidol with parenteral analgesics.
- Droperidol may aggravate symptoms of acute depression.

ENOXAPARIN

Class: Anticoagulant

Trade Name: Lovenox

Therapeutic Action/Pharmacodynamics: Enoxaparin is a low-molecular-weight heparin derivative that accelerates the formation of the antithrombin III-thrombin complex and deactivated thrombin, preventing the conversion of fibrinogen to fibrin. It is used primarily to prevent pulmonary embolism and deep vein thrombosis following hip and knee replacement surgery. Evidence also suggests that enoxaparin may be effective in the treatment of deep venous thrombosis and pulmonary embolism. It also can be used, in combination with oral aspirin, for patients with coronary ischemia associated with unstable angina and non-Q-wave myocardial infarction.

Emergency Uses: To inhibit clot formation in unstable angina and non-Q-wave myocardial infarction. *Adult dose:* 1 mg/kg SC.

To treat pulmonary embolism. *Adult dose:* 0.5 mg/kg IV.

Pharmacokinetics

Absorption: 92% absorbed; onset and peak within 3–5 hr; half-life is 4.5 hr.

Distribution: Preferential to the kidneys, liver, and spleen.

Excretion: Excreted in urine and breast milk.

Contraindications and Precautions: Enoxaparin is contraindicated in patients with a hypersensitivity to the drug, to pork products, and to heparin. Do not use in patients with active major bleeding or thrombocytopenia.

Adverse/Side Effects: CNS: Confusion, dizziness • CV: Edema, peripheral edema, chest pain, irregular heartbeat • GI: Nausea • Other: Irritation, pain, hematoma, or erythema at injection site, ecchymosis, bleeding complications, angioedema, rash, hives.

Interactions: NSAIDs, warfarin, antiplatelet agents (ticlopidine, dipyridamole) increase the risk of bleeding.

Prehospital Considerations
- Use with caution in the elderly and in any patients with an increased risk for bleeding, such as bacterial endocarditis, congenital bleeding disorders, ulcer disease, hemorrhagic stroke or recent brain or spinal surgery.
- Do not administer this drug IM.
- Do not massage the area following injection. Watch for signs of bleeding at site.

EPINEPHRINE

Class: Sympathomimetic

Trade Names: Adrenalin, Epinephrine

Therapeutic Action/Pharmacodynamics: Epinephrine is a naturally occurring catecholamine obtained from animal adrenal glands, but is also prepared synthetically. Acting directly on both alpha- and beta-adrenergic receptors, it is the most potent activator of alpha receptors. Epinephrine imitates all actions of the sympathetic nervous system except those on the arteries of the face and sweat glands. Its $beta_1$ effects strengthen myocardial contraction;

increase systolic but may decrease diastolic blood pressure; and increase cardiac rate and cardiac output. Its beta$_2$ effects dilate the bronchiole smooth muscle and inhibit mucus secretion that decreases overall airway resistance. Its alpha effects constrict the bronchial arterioles and inhibit histamine release, thus reducing congestion and edema and increasing tidal volume and vital capacity. Epinephrine also constricts arterioles, particularly in the skin, mucous membranes, and kidneys, but dilates skeletal muscle blood vessels. It relaxes uterine smooth musculature and inhibits uterine contractions. Its CNS actions are believed to result from peripheral effects.

Emergency Uses: To restore cardiac rhythm in cardiac arrest. *Adult dose:* 1 mg 1:10,000 IV every 3–5 min until circulation is restored. If given via ET tube, give 2.0–2.5 mg 1:10,000. *Pediatric dose:* 0.01 mg/kg 1:10,000 IV/IO. If given via ET, give 0.1 mg/kg of 1:1,000. All subsequent doses (IV/IO) at 0.1 mg/kg of 1:1,000.

For treatment of allergic reactions. *Adult dose:* 0.3–0.5 mg 1:1,000 SC or IM, every 5–15 min as needed; or 0.5–1.0 mg 1:10,000 IV if SC dose is ineffective or reaction severe. *Pediatric dose:* 0.01 mg/kg 1:1,000 SC or IM or 0.01 mg/kg of 1:10,000 IV every 10–15 min if SC dose is ineffective or reaction severe.

Pharmacokinetics
Absorption: Onset is less than 2 min IV, 3–10 min SC, less than 1 min ET; peak effect in less than 5 min IV/ET, 20 min SC; duration is 5–10 min IV/ET, 20–30 min SC.
Distribution: Widely distributed; does not cross blood-brain barrier; crosses placenta.
Metabolism: Metabolized in tissue and liver by MAO and COMT.
Elimination: Small amount excreted unchanged in urine; excreted in breast milk.

Contraindications and Precautions: There are no absolute contraindications to using epinephrine in cardiac arrest. In other cases, epinephrine is contraindicated in patients with a hypersensitivity to sympathomimetic amines; narrow-angle glaucoma; hemorrhagic, traumatic, or cardiogenic shock; cardiac dilatation, cerebral arteriosclerosis, coronary insufficiency, dysrhythmias, organic heart or brain disease; during second stage of labor. Safe use during pregnancy (category C), in nursing women, and in children is not established. Use with caution in the elderly or debilitated patients; hypertension; diabetes mellitus; hyperthyroidism; Parkinson's disease; tuberculosis; in patients with long-standing bronchial asthma and emphysema with degenerative heart disease; in children less than 6 yr of age.

Adverse/Side Effects: CNS: Nervousness, restlessness, sleeplessness, fear, anxiety, tremors, severe headache, cerebrovascular accident, weakness, dizziness, syncope • CV: Precordial pain, palpitations, hypertension, MI, tachydysrhythmias including ventricular fibrillation • GI: Nausea, vomiting • Skin: Pallor, sweating, tissue necrosis with repeated injections.

Interactions: Epinephrine may increase hypotension in circulatory collapse or hypotension caused by phenothiazines. It has additive toxicities with other sympathomimetics. Alpha- and beta-adrenergic blocking agents antagonize the effects of epinephrine. Epinephrine is pH dependent and can be deactivated when administered with highly alkaline solutions such as bicarbonate.

Prehospital Considerations
- A tuberculin syringe may ensure greater accuracy in measurement of parenteral doses.
- Epinephrine injection should be protected from exposure to light at all times. Do not remove ampule or vial from carton until ready to use.

- Carefully aspirate before injecting epinephrine. Inadvertent IV injection of usual SC doses can result in sudden hypertension and possibly cerebral hemorrhage.
- Vascular constriction from repeated injections may cause tissue necrosis. Rotate injection sites and observe for signs of blanching.
- For IV use in cardiac resuscitation, if the 1:1,000 1-mL ampules are used, the dose should be further diluted with 10 mL of sodium chloride injection.
- As a maintenance infusion, dilute in 500 mL 5% dextrose.
- IV administration: Give each 1 mg over 1 min or longer; may give more rapidly in cardiac arrest.
- Isoproterenol should not be used concurrently with epinephrine. A 4-hr interval should elapse before a change is made from one drug to the other.

EPTIFIBATIDE

Classes: IIb–IIIa glycoprotein inhibitor; antithrombotic; antiplatelet

Trade Name: Integrilin

Therapeutic Action/Pharmacodynamics: Eptifibatide binds to the IIb–IIIa glycoprotein receptors found on platelets and vessel wall endothelial and smooth muscle cells. This inhibits platelet aggregation by preventing fibrinogen and other adhesive molecules from binding with receptors on activated platelets.

Emergency Uses: Treatment of acute coronary syndromes (unstable angina, non-Q-wave MI) and patients undergoing percutaneous coronary interventions (PCIs). *Adult dose:* Dosing based on dosage chart (see drug insert).

Always used in combination with aspirin and heparin in acute coronary syndrome. *Pediatric dose:* Not indicated.

Pharmacokinetics
Absorption: Immediately absorbed; duration of 6–8 hr after stopping infusion, half-life is 2.5 hr.
Distribution: 25% protein bound.
Metabolism: Minimally metabolized.
Elimination: 50% excreted in urine.

Contraindications and Precautions: Because eptifibatide may increase the risk of bleeding, it is contraindicated in the following clinical situations: active internal bleeding; recent (within 6 wk) GI or GU bleeding of clinical significance; history of stroke within 2 yr or stroke with a significant residual neurologic deficit; thrombocytopenia; recent (within 6 wk) major surgery or trauma; intracranial neoplasm, arteriovenous malformation, or aneurysm; severe uncontrolled hypertension; presumed or documented history of vasculitis.

Adverse/Side Effects: CNS: Intracranial bleeding • GI/GU: Bleeding • Heme: Bleeding, anemia, thrombocytopenia.

Interactions: Oral anticoagulants, NSAIDs, dipyridamole, ticlopidine, dextran may increase risk of bleeding.

Prehospital Considerations
- Monitor for signs and symptoms of bleeding at all potential sites (e.g., catheter insertion, needle puncture; GI, GU, or retroperitoneal sites); hypersensitivity that may occur any time during administration.
- Avoid or minimize unnecessary invasive procedures and devices to reduce risk of bleeding.
- If symptoms of an allergic reaction or anaphylaxis appear, stop the infusion immediately and give the appropriate treatment.
- Although no incompatibilities have been shown with IV infusion fluids or commonly used cardiovascular drugs,

Eptifibatide

administer eptifibatide in a separate IV line whenever possible and not mixed with other medications.

ESMOLOL

Class: Beta blocker

Trade Name: Brevibloc

Therapeutic Action/Pharmacodynamics: Esmolol is an ultra-short-acting beta$_1$-adrenergic blocking agent with cardioselective properties but devoid of intrinsic sympathetic activity or membrane-stabilizing (quinidine-like) activity. Its hemodynamic effects are mild, with potency as a beta blocker about 1/100th that of propranolol. By competitive binding at beta-adrenergic receptors, it inhibits the agonist effect of catecholamines. Since it binds predominantly to beta$_1$-receptors in cardiac tissue, sympathetically mediated increases in cardiac rate and BP are blocked.

Emergency Use: To convert supraventricular tachydysrhythmias accompanied by a rapid ventricular response. *Adult dose:* Loading dose is 500 mcg/kg/min IV for 1 min. Maintenance dose is 50 mcg/kg/min IV for 4 min. If unsuccessful, repeat loading dose every 4 min and increase maintenance dose by 50 mcg/kg/min until desired effect is reached. Do not exceed maintenance dose of 300 mcg/kg/min.

Pharmacokinetics

Absorption: Onset is within 5 min; peak effect in 10–20 min; duration is 10–30 min; half-life is 9 min.
Metabolism: Rapidly hydrolyzed by RBC esterases.
Elimination: Eliminated in urine.

Contraindications and Precautions: Esmolol is contraindicated in cardiac failure, heart block greater than first degree, sinus bradycardia, and cardiogenic shock. Safe use during pregnancy (category C), in nursing mothers, and in children is not established. Use with caution in patients with a history of allergy or bronchial asthma, bronchospasm, emphysema; CHF; diabetes mellitus; renal function impairment.

Adverse/Side Effects: CNS: Headache, dizziness, somnolence, confusion, agitation • CV: Hypotension (dose related), cold hands and feet, bradydysrhythmias, flushing, myocardial depression • GI: Nausea, vomiting • Respiratory: Dyspnea, chest pain, rhonchi, bronchospasm • Skin: Infusion site inflammation (redness, swelling).

Interactions: Esmolol may increase digoxin levels 10–20%. IV morphine may increase esmolol levels by 45%; succinylcholine may prolong neuromuscular blockade. Never administer esmolol to patients receiving IV calcium channel blockers because profound hypotension may occur.

Prehospital Considerations
- Esmolol must be diluted before administration (available as a solution: 250 mg/mL in 10-mL ampules). Dilute each 5 g with 500 mL of D_5W, NS, or other appropriate diluent (see manufacturer's directions). Resulting solution yields 10 mg/mL. Caution: A stronger solution (e.g., 20 mg/mL) may cause venous irritation and thrombophlebitis.
- Do not admix with other drugs before dilution in a suitable IV fluid.
- The diluted infusion solution is stable for at least 24 hr at room temperature.
- Monitor BP, pulse, ECG during esmolol infusion.
- Hypotension may have its onset during the initial titration phase; thereafter the risk increases with increasing doses.

Esmolol

85

Usually the hypotension experienced during esmolol infusion is resolved within 30 min after infusion is reduced or discontinued.

- IV site reactions (burning, erythema) or diaphoresis may develop during infusion. Both reactions are temporary, but injection site should be changed if local reaction occurs. Blood chemistry abnormalities have not been reported.
- Overdose symptoms: Discontinue administration if the following symptoms occur: bradycardia, severe dizziness or drowsiness, dyspnea, bluish-colored fingernails or palms of hands, seizures.

ETOMIDATE

Class: Hypnotic

Trade Name: Amidate

Therapeutic Action/Pharmacodynamics: Etomidate is an ultra-short-acting, nonbarbiturate hypnotic, with no analgesic effects, used for facilitated intubation. It produces a rapid induction of anesthesia with minimal cardiovascular and respiratory effects. It is rapidly distributed following IV injection or infusion and rapidly metabolized and excreted. Etomidate has advantages over other short-acting induction anesthetics, particularly barbiturates, in that it does not cause histamine release; its effects on the cardiovascular and respiratory systems are minimal, and there are no reports of organ toxicity or biochemical or hematological disturbances. Its short duration of action and relative safety make it an effective drug to induce sedation for facilitated intubation.

Emergency Use: To induce sedation for endotracheal intubation. *Adult dose:* 0.1–0.3 mg/kg IV over 15–30 sec. *Pediatric dose:* Children older than 10 yr, same as for adult.

Pharmacokinetics

Absorption: Onset in 10–20 sec, peak effects within 1 min; duration is 3–5 min; half-life is 30–74 min.

Metabolism: Rapidly metabolized in the liver with inactive metabolites.

Elimination: Excreted mainly through the urine.

Contraindications and Precautions: Etomidate is contraindicated in patients with a hypersensitivity to the drug. Use with caution in patients with marked hypotension, severe asthma, or severe cardiovascular disease. Its safety in children under 10 yr has not been established.

Adverse/Side Effects: CNS: Myoclonic skeletal muscle movements, tonic movements • Respiratory: Apnea, hyperventilation or hypoventilation, laryngospasm • CV: Either hypertension or hypotension; tachycardia or bradycardia; dysrhythmias • GI: Nausea, vomiting • Miscellaneous: Eye movements (common), hiccups, snoring.

Interactions: None in the emergency setting.

Prehospital Considerations

- Verapamil may cause prolonged respiratory depression and apnea.
- It is important to remember that etomidate does not have any analgesic properties. Thus, an analgesic should be administered with etomidate for painful procedures such as electrical cardioversion.
- Nausea is common following recovery from etomidate. This side effect should be expected and treated accordingly.
- Myotonic jerks are also common following etomidate administration. Although benign, these jerks can cause pain in patients with injuries such as long bone fractures.
- Flumazenil DOES NOT reverse the effects of etomidate.

Etomidate

FENTANYL CITRATE

Class: Narcotic analgesic

Trade Name: Sublimaze

Therapeutic Action/Pharmacodynamics: Fentanyl is a potent synthetic narcotic agonist analgesic with pharmacologic actions qualitatively similar to those of morphine and meperidine, but whose action is quicker and less prolonged. Its principal actions are analgesia and sedation. Drug-induced alterations in respiratory rate and alveolar ventilation may persist beyond the analgesic effect. The emetic effect is less than with either morphine or meperidine.

Emergency Uses: To induce sedation during rapid-sequence intubation procedure; to control severe pain. *Adult dose:* 25–100 mcg slow IV (over 2–3 min). *Pediatric dose:* 2.0 mcg/kg slow IV/IM.

Pharmacokinetics

Absorption: Onset is immediate; peak effect in 3–5 min IV; duration is 30–60 min.

Metabolism: Metabolized in liver.

Elimination: Excreted in urine.

Contraindications and Precautions: Fentanyl is contraindicated in patients who have received MAO inhibitors within 14 days; myasthenia gravis. Safe use during pregnancy (category C) and in children under 2 yr is not established. Use with caution in head injuries, increased intracranial pressure; elderly, debilitated, or poor-risk patients; COPD, other respiratory problems; liver and kidney dysfunction; bradydysrhythmias.

Adverse/Side Effects: CNS: Sedation, euphoria, dizziness, diaphoresis, delirium, convulsions with high doses • CV: Hypotension, bradycardia, circulatory depression, cardiac arrest • Eye: Miosis, blurred vision • GI: Nausea, vomiting, constipation, ileus • Respiratory: Laryngospasm, bronchoconstriction, respiratory depression or arrest • Other: Muscle rigidity, especially muscles of respiration after rapid IV infusion, urinary retention, rash.

Interactions: Alcohol and other CNS depressants potentiate its effects; MAO inhibitors may precipitate hypertensive crisis.

Prehospital Considerations

- Parenteral doses may be given undiluted or diluted in 5 mL sterile water or NS. Administer by direct IV over 1–2 min.
- Store at 15–30C (59–86F) unless otherwise directed. Protect drug from light.
- Monitor vital signs and observe patient for signs of skeletal and thoracic muscle (depressed respirations) rigidity and weakness.
- Duration of respiratory depressant effect may be considerably longer than narcotic analgesic effect. Have immediately available oxygen, resuscitative and intubation equipment, and an opioid antagonist such as naloxone.

FLECAINIDE

Class: Antidysrhythmic

Trade Name: Tambocor

Therapeutic Action/Pharmacodynamics: Flecainide is a local (membrane) anesthetic and antidysrhythmic with electrophysiologic properties similar to other class IC antidysrhythmic drugs. It slows conduction velocity throughout the myocardial conduction system and increases ventricular refractoriness but has little effect on repolarization. Flecainide prolongs the His-ventricular

(HQ) and QRS intervals at therapeutic doses. Clinically, flecainide causes both hypotension and negative inotropy (in higher dose ranges) and is an effective suppressant of PVCs and a variety of atrial and ventricular arrhythmias.

Emergency Uses: To convert atrial flutter and atrial fibrillation, AV nodal reentrant tachycardia, and SVT associated with Wolff-Parkinson-White syndrome. *Adult dose:* 100 mg PO every 12 hr; may increase by 50 mg twice a day every 4 days to a maximum of 400 mg/day. IV dose is 2 mg/kg administered at 10 mg/min. *Pediatric dose:* 1–3 mg/kg/day PO in 3 divided doses (maximum 8 mg/kg/day).

Pharmacokinetics
Absorption: Readily absorbed from GI tract; peak effect in 2–3 hr; half-life is 7–22 hr.
Distribution: Crosses placenta; distributed into breast milk.
Metabolism: Metabolized in liver.
Elimination: Excreted mainly in urine.

Contraindications and Precautions: Flecainide is contraindicated in patients with a hypersensitivity to flecainide; preexisting second- or third-degree AV block, right bundle branch block when associated with a left hemiblock unless a pacemaker is present; cardiogenic shock, significant hepatic impairment. Use with caution in patients with CHF, sick sinus syndrome, and renal impairment.

Adverse/Side Effects: CNS: Dizziness, headache, light-headedness, unsteadiness, paresthesias, fatigue • CV: Arrhythmias, chest pain, worsening of CHF • Eye: Blurred vision, difficulty in focusing, and spots before eyes • GI: Nausea, constipation, change in taste perception • Other: Dyspnea, fever, and edema.

Interactions: Cimetidine may increase flecainide levels; may increase digoxin levels 15–25%; beta blockers may have additive negative inotropic effects.

Prehospital Considerations

- IV use of flecainide is not approved in the United States.
- Avoid using flecainide in patients who have had MI, because of its negative inotropic effects. It has been observed to increase mortality.
- Flecainide is limited by its need to be infused slowly, which may make it impractical for emergency medicine.
- Dosage increases more frequently than every 4 days are not recommended.
- Store in tightly covered, light-resistant containers at 15–30C (59–86F) unless otherwise directed.
- ECG monitoring is essential because of the possibility of drug-induced arrhythmias.
- Once arrhythmia is controlled, dosage reduction may be attempted with caution.
- Impress on patient the importance of taking drug at the prescribed times.
- Instruct patient to report visual disturbances.
- Instruct patient to report immediately passage of dark, tarry stools, "coffee ground" emesis, frank bloody emesis, or other GI distress.
- Advise patient to report immediately to physician the onset of skin rash, pruritus, jaundice.
- Inform patients about possible CNS effects (light-headedness, dizziness, drowsiness) and caution them to avoid dangerous activities until reaction to the drug has been determined.
- Patients should avoid self-medication with ibuprofen if taking prescribed drugs or if being treated for a serious condition without consulting physician.
- Patients should avoid taking aspirin or acetaminophen concurrently with ibuprofen.
- Inform patient that alcohol and NSAIDs may increase risk of GI ulceration and bleeding tendencies and should be avoided, unless otherwise advised by physician.

FLUMAZENIL

Class: Benzodiazepine antagonist

Trade Name: Romazicon

Therapeutic Action/Pharmacodynamics: Flumazenil antagonizes the sedative effects of benzodiazepines in the central nervous system (sedation, impairment of recall, and psychomotor impairment) by inhibiting their effects on the GABA/benzodiazepine complex. Flumazenil is used to reverse the respiratory depression caused by the following drugs: diazepam (Valium), midazolam (Versed), lorazepam (Ativan), triazolam (Halcion), temazepam (Restoril), zolpidem (Ambien), flurazepam (Dalmane), clorazepate (Tranxene), oxazepam (Serax), clonazepam (Klonopin), quazepam (Doral), estazolam (ProSom), alprazolam (Xanax). It does not reverse the effects of opioids.

Emergency Use: To reverse the respiratory depression caused by benzodiazepines. *Adult dose:* 0.2 mg IV over 30 sec. May be repeated up to 1 mg.

Pharmacokinetics

Absorption: Onset in 1–5 min; peak effect in 6–10 min; duration is 2–4 hr; half-life is 54 min.

Metabolism: Metabolized in the liver to inactive metabolites.

Elimination: 90–95% excreted in urine, 5–10% in feces within 72 hr.

Contraindications and Precautions: Flumazenil should not be used as a diagnostic agent for benzodiazepine overdose in the same manner that naloxone is used for narcotic overdose. The potential for inducing a life-threatening withdrawal reaction in patients addicted to benzodiazepines with flumazenil is not worth the perceived benefits. It is contraindicated in patients with a hypersensitivity to flumazenil or to benzodiazepines; patients given a benzodiazepine for control of a life-threatening condition (such as status epilepticus); patients showing signs of tricyclic anti-depressant overdose; seizure-prone individuals during labor and delivery. Its effects on children are unknown. Use with caution in patients with hepatic function impairment, the elderly, pregnancy (category C), nursing mothers, intensive care patients, head injury, drug- and alcohol-dependent patients, and physical dependence upon benzodiazepines.

Adverse/Side Effects: CNS: Emotional instability, headache, dizziness, agitation, resedation, seizures, blurred vision • GI: Nausea, vomiting, hiccups • Other: Shivering, pain at injection site, hypoventilation.

Interactions: Few in the emergency setting.

Prehospital Considerations

- Ensure patency of IV before administration of flumazenil, since extravasation will cause local irritation.
- Flumazenil should be administered through an IV that is freely flowing into a large vein.
- Flumazenil should not be administered as a bolus dose; instead, each 0.2-mg dose should be given in small quantities over 15 sec. Doses of flumazenil are given at 60-sec intervals.
- In high-risk patients, slow the rate of administration of flumazenil to intervals of 6–10 min to provide the smallest effective dose.
- If resedation occurs, repeat doses may be given at 20-min intervals. Maximum dose for repeat treatment is 1 mg given at a rate of 0.2 mg/min, not to exceed 3 mg in any 1-hr period.
- Monitor patients for reversal of benzodiazepine for up to 120 min for respiratory depression and resedation.
- Benzodiazepine-induced ventilatory insufficiency may not be fully reversed by flumazenil; carefully monitor respiratory status until risk of resedation is unlikely.

- Monitor carefully for seizures and take appropriate precautions.
- Seizures induced by flumazenil administration probably will not respond to treatment with a benzodiazepine. Instead, antiseizure drugs from another class, such as phenytoin or phenobarbital, must be used.

FOSPHENYTOIN

Class: Anticonvulsant

Trade Name: Cerebyx

Therapeutic Action/Pharmacodynamics: Fosphenytoin is a prodrug of phenytoin. Following administration, fosphenytoin is converted to the anticonvulsant phenytoin. The cellular mechanisms of phenytoin are thought to be responsible for fosphenytoin's anticonvulsant effects. Fosphenytoin is thought to modulate the sodium channels of neurons, modulate calcium flux across neuronal membranes, and enhance the sodium-potassium ATPase activity of neurons and glial cells.

Emergency Uses: Fosphenytoin is used to control seizures, especially status epilepticus, and to prevent seizures in seizure-prone patients. *Adult dose:* IV loading dose of 15–20 mg PE/kg administered at 100–150 mg PE/min. Initial maintenance dose is 4–6 mg PE/kg/day. All fosphenytoin doses are expressed in phenytoin sodium equivalents (PE) to simplify calculations between phenytoin and fosphenytoin.

Pharmacokinetics

Absorption: Completely absorbed after IV/IM administration; peak effect in 30 min IM.

Distribution: 95–99% protein bound. Crosses placenta, distributed into breast milk.

Metabolism: Extensively metabolized in the liver via oxidation.

Elimination: Phenytoin excreted in urine as metabolites.

Contraindications and Precautions: Fosphenytoin is contraindicated in patients with hypersensitivity to the drug, seizures due to hypoglycemia, sinus bradycardia, complete or incomplete heart block, Stokes-Adams syndrome, pregnancy (category D), lactation. Use with caution in patients with impaired hepatic or renal function, alcoholism, hypotension, heart block, bradycardia, severe CAD, diabetes mellitus, hyperglycemia, and respiratory depression.

Adverse/Side Effects: CNS: Usually dose-related: paresthesias, tinnitus, nystagmus, dizziness, drowsiness, confusion, and tremors • CV: Arrhythmias, hypotension, hypertension, cardiovascular collapse • GI: Nausea, vomiting, dysphagia • Eye: Conjunctivitis, photophobia, diplopia • Metabolic: Fever, hyperglycemia • Other: Rash, acute renal failure.

Interactions: Alcohol decreases fosphenytoin effects. Amiodarone, chloramphenicol, and omperazole increase fosphenytoin levels.

Prehospital Considerations
- Fosphenytoin may be administered IM in addition to IV.
- IV fosphenytoin should be diluted in D_5W or NS.
- Closely monitor ECG, pulse, blood pressure, and respiratory function during administration.
- Discontinue infusion if rash appears.
- Carefully monitor for adverse effects.
- Fosphenytoin costs considerably more than phenytoin.

FUROSEMIDE

Class: Loop diuretic

Trade Names: Apo-Furosemide (Can), Furoside (Can), Lasix, Novo-Semide (Can), Urex (Aus), Uritrol (Can)

Therapeutic Action/Pharmacodynamics: Furosemide is a rapid-acting potent sulfonamide loop diuretic and antihypertensive with pharmacologic effects and uses almost identical to those of ethacrynic acid. Its exact mode of action is not clearly defined. Renal vascular resistance decreases, and renal blood flow may increase during drug administration. It inhibits reabsorption of sodium and chloride primarily in the loop of Henle and also in proximal and distal renal tubules. It is reportedly less ototoxic than ethacrynic acid. Its venodilating effect reduces cardiac preload, which decreases the cardiac workload.

Emergency Uses: To treat acute pulmonary edema and congestive heart failure. *Adult dose:* 40–120 mg slow IV. *Pediatric dose:* 1 mg/kg slow IV.

Pharmacokinetics

Absorption: Onset of vasodilation is 5–10 min; diuresis is 5–30 min. Peak vasodilatory effect in 30 min; peak diuresis in 20–60 min. Vasodilatory duration is less than 2 hr; diuresis duration is 6 hr; half-life is 30 min.
Metabolism: Small amount metabolized in liver.
Elimination: Rapidly excreted in urine; 80% of IV dose excreted within 24 hr; excreted in breast milk.

Contraindications and Precautions: Furosemide is contraindicated in patients with a history of hypersensitivity to furosemide or sulfonamides; increasing oliguria, anuria, fluid and electrolyte depletion states; hepatic coma; pregnancy (category C). Use with caution in infants, elderly patients; hepatic cirrhosis, nephrotic syndrome; cardiogenic shock associated with acute MI, history of gout; patients receiving digitalis glycosides or potassium-depleting steroids.

Adverse/Side Effects: CV: Postural hypotension, dizziness with excessive diuresis, acute hypotensive episodes, circulatory collapse • Fluid and electrolyte imbalance: Hypovolemia, dehydration, hyponatremia, hypokalemia, hypochloremia metabolic alkalosis, hypomagnesemia, hypocalcemia (tetany) • GI: Nausea, vomiting, oral and gastric burning, anorexia, diarrhea, constipation, abdominal cramping, acute pancreatitis, jaundice • GU: Allergic interstitial nephritis, irreversible renal failure, urinary frequency • Hematologic: Anemia, leukopenia, thrombocytopenic purpura • Rare: Aplastic anemia, agranulocytosis • Ototoxicity: Tinnitus, vertigo, feeling of fullness in ears, hearing loss (rarely permanent) • Skin: Pruritus, urticaria, exfoliative dermatitis, purpura, photosensitivity • Other: Hyperglycemia, glycosuria, elevated BUN, hyperuricemia; increased perspiration; paresthesias; blurred vision, muscle spasms, weakness; thrombophlebitis, pain at IM injection site.

Interactions: Other diuretics enhance the diuretic effects of furosemide. There is an increased risk of digoxin toxicity because of hypokalemia. Nondepolarizing neuromuscular blocking agents (e.g., tubocurarine) prolong neuromuscular blockage. Corticosteroids can potentiate hypokalemia. Furosemide decreases lithium elimination and increases its toxicity; it blunts the hypoglycemic effects of insulin. NSAIDs may attenuate diuretic effects.

Prehospital Considerations

- Protect syringes from light once they are removed from package.
- IV administration: IV furosemide may be given by direct IV undiluted at a rate of 20 mg or a fraction thereof over 1 min. With high doses a rate of 4 mg/min is recommended to decrease risk of ototoxicity.
- IV administration to neonates, infants, children: Verify correct IV concentration and rate of infusion/injection with physician.
- Infusion solutions in which furosemide has been mixed should be used within 24 hr.

Furosemide

- Patients receiving the drug parenterally should be observed carefully, and BP and vital signs closely monitored. Sudden death from cardiac arrest has been reported.
- Close observation of the elderly patient is particularly essential during period of brisk diuresis. Sudden alteration in fluid and electrolyte balance may precipitate significant adverse reactions. Report these symptoms to physician.
- Furosemide should not be administered through the same IV line as amrinone/inamrinone because it will cause a precipitate to form in the line.

GLUCAGON

Class: Hormone

Trade Name: GlucaGen

Therapeutic Action/Pharmacodynamics: Glucagon is a natural polypeptide hormone produced by alpha cells of the islets of Langerhans in the pancreas. When released it causes a breakdown of stored glycogen to glucose and inhibits the synthesis of glycogen from glucose. Both actions increase the blood levels of glucose. Given via the IM route, it is a useful drug in hypoglycemia when IV access is unsuccessful. Glucagon also increases heart rate and myocardial contractility and improves AV conduction in a manner similar to that produced by catecholamines. Its actions are independent of beta blockade.

Emergency Uses: To increase blood glucose levels in hypoglycemia without IV access. *Adult dose:* 1.0 mg IM/SC, may repeat every 5–20 min. *Pediatric dose:* 0.03–0.1 mg/kg/dose every 20 min as needed (maximum dose 1.0 mg).

To reverse the effects of beta blocker overdose. *Adult dose:* 50–150 mcg/kg IV over 1 min. *Pediatric dose:* 50–150 mcg/kg IV over 1 min. The literature supporting the use of glucagon in beta blocker overdose is extremely limited.

Pharmacokinetics

Absorption: Onset 5–20 min; peak effects in 30 min; duration is 1–1.5 hr; half-life is 3–10 min.
Metabolism: Metabolized in liver, plasma, and kidneys.
Elimination: Eliminated in urine.

Contraindications and Precautions: Glucagon is contraindicated in patients with a hypersensitivity to glucagon or protein compounds. Safe use during pregnancy (category B) and in nursing women is not established. Glucagon is effective only if there are glycogen stores in the liver. Use with caution in patients with a history of cardiovascular or renal disease.

Adverse/Side Effects: CNS: Dizziness, headache • CV: Hypotension • GI: Nausea and vomiting • Other: Hypersensitivity reactions, hyperglycemia, hypokalemia.

Interactions: None in the emergency setting.

Prehospital Considerations

- After reconstitution of dry powder, use solution immediately.
- Glucagon will form a precipitate in saline solutions and solutions with pH of 3–9.5 (pH of glucagon is 2.5–3). Glucagon should be considered incompatible in syringe with any other drug.
- Patient usually awakens from (diabetic) hypoglycemic coma 5–20 min after glucagon injection. As soon as possible after patient regains consciousness, PO carbohydrate should be given.
- After recovery from hypoglycemic reaction, symptoms such as headache, nausea, and weakness may persist.
- Most emergency departments and EMS services do not carry enough glucagon for a severe adult beta blocker overdose. A kit with an adequate quantity of the drug could be kept with a supervisor unit in case it is needed.

Glucagon

HALOPERIDOL

Class: Antipsychotic

Trade Names: Haldol, Peridol (Can), Serenace (Aus)

Therapeutic Action/Pharmacodynamics: Haloperidol is a potent, long-acting antipsychotic agent with pharmacologic actions similar to those of the phenothiazines but with a higher incidence of extrapyramidal effects and less hypotensive and relatively low sedative activity. While its exact mechanism is unclear, it appears to block the dopamine receptors in the brain associated with mood and behavior. It exerts strong antiemetic effects and impairs central thermoregulation. It also produces weak central anticholinergic effects and transient orthostatic hypotension.

Emergency Use: To manage acute psychotic disorders. *Adult dose:* 2–5 mg IM. *Pediatric dose:* 0.05–0.15 mg/kg/day PO in 2–3 divided doses.

Pharmacokinetics

Absorption: Onset in 30–45 min; peak effects in 10–20 min; half-life is 3–35 hr.

Distribution: Distributes mainly to liver with lower concentration in brain, lung, kidney, spleen, heart.

Metabolism: Metabolized in liver.

Elimination: 40% excreted in urine within 5 days; 15% eliminated in feces; excreted in breast milk.

Contraindications and Precautions: Haloperidol is contraindicated in Parkinson's disease, parkinsonism, seizure disorders, coma; alcoholism; severe mental depression, CNS depression; thyrotoxicosis. Safe use during pregnancy (category C), in nursing mothers, and in children under 3 yr is not established. Do not administer haloperidol if other sedatives have been given. Use with caution in elderly or debilitated patients or those with urinary retention, glaucoma, severe cardiovascular disorders;

in patients receiving anticonvulsant, anticoagulant, or lithium therapy.

Adverse/Side Effects: CNS: Extrapyramidal reactions: parkinsonism symptoms, dystonia, akathisia, tardive dyskinesia (after long-term use); insomnia, restlessness, anxiety, euphoria, agitation, drowsiness, mental depression, lethargy, fatigue, weakness, tremor, ataxia, headache, confusion, vertigo; neuroleptic malignant syndrome, hyperthermia, grand mal seizures, exacerbation of psychotic symptoms • CV: Tachycardia, ECG changes, hypotension, hypertension (with overdosage) • Endocrine: Menstrual irregularities, galactorrhea, lactation, gynecomastia, impotence, increased libido, hyponatremia, hyperglycemia, hypoglycemia • Eyes: Blurred vision • Hematologic: Mild transient leukopenia, agranulocytosis (rare) • GI: Dry mouth, anorexia, nausea, vomiting, constipation, diarrhea, hypersalivation • GU: Urinary retention, priapism • Respiratory: Laryngospasm, bronchospasm, increased depth of respiration, bronchopneumonia, respiratory depression • Skin: Diaphoresis, maculopapular and acneiform rash, photosensitivity • Other: Cholestatic jaundice, variations in liver function tests, decreased serum cholesterol.

Interactions: CNS depressants, opiates, and alcohol may increase CNS depression. Haloperidol may antagonize the activity of oral anticoagulants. Anticholinergics may increase intraocular pressure. Methyldopa may precipitate dementia.

Prehospital Considerations
- Haloperidol should be administered by deep IM injection into a large muscle. Do not exceed 3 mL per injection site.
- Have patient recumbent at time of parenteral administration and for about 1 hr after injection. Assess for orthostatic hypotension.

Haloperidol

- Dosing regimen should be tapered when therapy is to be discontinued. Abrupt termination can initiate extrapyramidal symptoms.
- Store in light-resistant container at 15–30C (59–86F), unless otherwise specified by manufacturer. Discard darkened solutions.
- Targeted symptoms expected to decrease with successful haloperidol treatment include hallucinations, insomnia, hostility, agitation, and delusions.
- Because of long half-life, therapeutic effects are slow to develop in early therapy or when established dosing regimen is changed.
- Therapeutic window effect (point at which increased dose or concentration actually decreases therapeutic response) may occur after long period of high doses. Close observation is imperative when doses are changed.
- In emergency situations where the patient's behavior poses an immediate risk to rescuers and bystanders, the initial IM injection may be given through the patient's clothing to minimize needle-stick injuries to rescuers.
- Extrapyramidal (EPS) or dystonic reactions are common with Haldol. Parenteral diphenhydramine (Benadryl) or benztropine (Cogentin) should be readily available.

HEPARIN

Class: Anticoagulant
Trade Names: Hepalean (Can), Heparin, Liquaemin Sodium, Uniparen (Aus)
Therapeutic Action/Pharmacodynamics: Heparin is a rapid-onset anticoagulant. It exerts direct effect on blood coagulation (clotting) by enhancing the inhibitory actions of antithrombin III (heparin cofactor) on several factors

essential to normal blood clotting, thereby blocking the conversion of prothrombin to thrombin and fibrinogen to fibrin. Heparin does not lyse already existing thrombi but may prevent their extension and propagation. It also inhibits formation of new clots.

Emergency Use: To prevent thrombus formation in acute MI. *Adult dose:* 5,000 U IV, then 20,000–40,000 U IV over 24 hr.

Pharmacokinetics

Onset: Immediate onset; peak effect within minutes; duration is 2–6 hr; half-life is 90 min.
Distribution: Does not cross placenta; not distributed into breast milk.
Metabolism: Metabolized in liver and by reticuloendothelial system.
Elimination: Excreted slowly in urine.

Contraindications and Precautions: Heparin is contraindicated in patients with a history of hypersensitivity to the drug, active bleeding, and bleeding tendencies (hemophilia, purpura, thrombocytopenia). Use with caution in alcoholism; history of atopy or allergy (asthma, hives, hay fever, eczema); during menstruation, pregnancy (category C), especially the last trimester, and immediate postpartum period; patients with indwelling catheters; the elderly; patients in hazardous occupations; cerebral embolism.

Adverse/Side Effects: CNS: Numbness and tingling of hands and feet, headache • CV: Spontaneous bleeding, cyanosis and pains in arms or legs (vasospasm), hypertension, chest pain • Respiratory: Nasal congestion, bronchospasm • Skin: Injection site reactions: pain, itching, ecchymoses, tissue irritation and sloughing, urticaria, pruritus, skin rashes, itching and burning sensations of feet.

Heparin

Interactions: Aspirin and other NSAIDs increase risk of bleeding. Nitroglycerin IV may decrease anticoagulant activity. Protamine antagonizes effects of heparin.

Prehospital Considerations

- A single dose of IV heparin (adult 5,000 U, child 50 U/kg) may be given undiluted by direct IV injection over 60 sec.
- IV heparin may be added to NS, D_5W, or Ringer's for injection and infused intermittently or continuously. When heparin is added to an infusion solution, invert container at least 6 times to ensure adequate mixing.
- Continuous IV infusion of heparin requires a constant-infusion pump.
- Patients vary widely in their reaction to heparin. The risk of hemorrhage appears to be greatest in women, all patients over 60 yr, and patients with liver disease or renal insufficiency.
- Monitor vital signs. Report fever, drop in BP, rapid pulse and other signs of hemorrhage.
- A dilute heparin solution may be used to flush IV catheters (heparin locks) to prevent clotting.

HYDRALAZINE

Class: Antihypertensive

Trade Names: Alphapress (Aus), Apresoline, Novo-Hylazin (Can), Supres (Can)

Therapeutic Action/Pharmacodynamics: Hydralazine reduces blood pressure mainly by direct effect on vascular smooth muscles, resulting in vasodilation. It has little effect on venous-capacitance vessels. The diastolic response is often greater than systolic. Vasodilation reduces preload and substantially improves cardiac output, and renal and cerebral blood flow. Its hypotensive effects may be limited by sympathetic reflexes, which increase heart rate, stroke volume, and cardiac output. The postural hypotensive effect is reportedly less than that produced by sodium nitroprusside.

Emergency Uses: To reduce blood pressure in hypertensive crisis and preeclampsia. *Adult dose:* 20–40 mg IV/IM. May be repeated in 4–6 hr. *Pediatric dose:* 0.1–0.5 mg/kg/day IV/IM.

Pharmacokinetics

Absorption: Onset is 5–15 min IV, 10–40 min IM; peak effects in less than 80 min; duration is 2–6 hr; half-life is 2–8 hr.
Distribution: Crosses placenta; distributed into breast milk.
Metabolism: Metabolized in intestinal wall and liver.
Elimination: 90% rapidly excreted in urine; 10% excreted in feces.

Contraindications and Precautions: Hydralazine is contraindicated in patients with a hypersensitivity to the drug, coronary artery disease, or mitral valvular rheumatic heart disease, MI, tachycardia, SLE. Safe use during pregnancy (category C) or in nursing mothers is not established. Use with caution in patients with cerebrovascular accident, advanced renal impairment, and those taking MAO inhibitors.

Adverse/Side Effects: CNS: Headache, dizziness, tremors • CV: Palpitation, angina, tachycardia, flushing, paradoxical pressor response, dysrhythmia, shock • Eye: Lacrimation, conjunctivitis • GI: Anorexia, nausea, vomiting, diarrhea, constipation, abdominal pain, paralytic ileus • GU: Difficulty in urination, glomerulonephritis • Hematologic: Decreased hematocrit and hemoglobin, anemia • Hypersensitivity: Rash, urticaria, pruritus, fever, chills, arthralgia, eosinophilia, cholangitis, hepatitis, obstructive jaundice • Other: Nasal congestion, muscle cramps, edema.

Hydralazine

Interactions: Beta blockers and other antihypertensive agents compound the hypotensive effects.

Prehospital Considerations

- Administer undiluted solution by direct IV. Give each 10 mg or fraction thereof over 1 min. Do not add hydralazine to IV solutions.
- Discontinuation of hydralazine should be accomplished gradually to avoid sudden rise in BP and acute heart failure. Patients should be informed of the dangers of abrupt withdrawal.
- Store at 15–30C (59–86F) in tight, light-resistant containers unless otherwise directed. Avoid freezing.
- Closely monitor BP and heart rate. Check every 5 min until it is stabilized at desired level, then every 15 min thereafter throughout hypertensive crisis.

HYDROCORTISONE

Class: Steroid

Trade Name: Solu-Cortef

Therapeutic Action/Pharmacodynamics: Hydrocortisone is a short-acting synthetic steroid with both glucocorticoid and mineralocorticoid properties that affect nearly all systems of the body. By inhibiting the formation, storage, and release of histamine from mast cells, it reduces the effects of an allergic response. It also increases the body's response to circulating catecholamines.

Emergency Uses: To reduce inflammation during an allergic reaction, severe anaphylaxis, asthma, or COPD; to treat urticaria. *Adult dose:* 40–250 mg IV/IM. *Pediatric dose:* 4–8 mg/kg/IM/IV.

Pharmacokinetics

Absorption: Onset is immediate; peak effect in 4–8 hr; duration is 1–1.5 days; half-life is 90 min.

Distribution: Distributed primarily to muscles, liver, skin, intestines, kidneys; crosses placenta.

Metabolism: Metabolized in the liver.

Elimination: Metabolites excreted in urine; excreted in breast milk.

Contraindications and Precautions: Hydrocortisone is contraindicated in patients with hypersensitivity to gluco-corticoids. In the treatment of anaphylaxis, there are no absolute contraindications. In the prehospital phase of care, give only a single bolus. Long-term steroid therapy can cause gastrointestinal bleeding, prolonged wound healing, and suppression of the adrenocortical steroids.

Adverse/Side Effects: CNS: Vertigo, headache, nystagmus, ataxia (rare), increased intracranial pressure with papilledema (usually after discontinuation of medication), mental disturbances, aggravation of preexisting psychiatric conditions, insomnia • CV: Syncopal episodes, throm-bophlebitis, thromboembolism or fat embolism, palpitation, tachycardia, necrotizing angiitis • Endocrine: Decreased glucose tolerance; hyperglycemia, manifestations of latent diabetes mellitus; hypocorticism; amenorrhea and other menstrual difficulties • Eye: Posterior subcapsular cataracts (especially in children), glaucoma, exophthalmos, increased intraocular pressure with optic nerve damage, perforation of the globe, fungal infection of the cornea, decreased or blurred vision • Fluid and electrolyte disturbances: Hypocalcemia; sodium and fluid retention; hypokalemia and hypokalemic alkalosis; CHF, hypertension • GI: Nausea, increased appetite, ulcerative esophagitis, pancreatitis, abdominal distension, peptic ulcer with perforation and hemorrhage, melena • Hematologic: Thrombocytopenia • Musculoskeletal (long-term use): Osteoporosis, compression fractures, muscle wasting and weakness, tendon rupture, aseptic necrosis of femoral and humeral heads • Skin: Skin thinning and atrophy, acne, impaired wound healing; petechiae, ecchymosis, easy bruising; suppression of skin test reaction; hypopigmentation or hyperpigmentation, hirsutism, acneiform eruptions, subcutaneous fat atrophy; allergic dermatitis, urticaria, angioneurotic edema, increased sweating • Other: Hypersensitivity or anaphylactoid reactions; aggravation or masking of infections; malaise, weight gain, obesity; decreased serum concentration of vitamins A and C; urinary frequency and urgency, enuresis • Overdose: Anxiety, mental confusion, depression, hyperglycemia, hypokalemia, hypernatremia, polycythemia, hypertension, edema, GI cramping or bleeding, ecchymoses • With parenteral therapy: IV site: pain, irritation, necrosis, atrophy, sterile abscess; Charcot-like arthropathy following intra-articular use; burning and tingling in perineal area (after IV injection).

Interactions: Barbiturates, phenytoin, and rifampin may increase hepatic metabolism, thus decreasing cortisone levels. Estrogens may potentiate the effects of hydrocortisone. NSAIDs compound its ulcerogenic effects. Diuretics, amphotericin B exacerbate hypokalemia; anticholinesterase agents (e.g., neostigmine) may produce severe weakness; immune response to vaccines and toxoids may be decreased.

Prehospital Considerations

- Inject IM preparation deep into gluteal muscle.
- IV administration: IV hydrocortisone may be given by direct IV undiluted or diluted in NS or D_5W. Administer at a rate of 25 mg or a fraction thereof over 1 min.
- IV administration to infants, children: Verify correct IV concentration and rate of infusion/injection with physician.
- Solutions that have been diluted for IV infusion should be administered within 24 hr of dilution.
- The elderly and the patient with low serum albumin are especially susceptible to adverse or side effects.

HYDROXYZINE

Class: Antihistamine

Trade Names: Anxanil, Atarax, Hydroxacin, Multipax (Can), Quiess, Vistaject, Vistaril

Therapeutic Action/Pharmacodynamics: Hydroxyzine is an antihistamine with CNS depressive, sedative, anticholinergic, antiemetic, and bronchodilator properties. Its tranquilizing (ataractic) effect is produced primarily by depression of hypothalamus and brain-stem reticular formation, rather than cortical areas. It is used frequently in the emergency setting, often in combination with analgesics.

Emergency Uses: To manage an acute anxiety attack. *Adult dose:* 50–100 mg deep IM. *Pediatric dose:* 1 mg/kg IM.

To control nausea and vomiting. *Adult dose:* 25–50 mg deep IM. *Pediatric dose:* 1 mg/kg deep IM.

Pharmacokinetics

Absorption: Onset is 15–30 min; duration is 4–6 hr.
Distribution: Not known if it crosses placenta or is distributed into breast milk.
Metabolism: Metabolized in liver.
Elimination: Probably excreted in bile.

Contraindications and Precautions: Hydroxyzine is contraindicated in patients with known hypersensitivity to the drug. Safe use during pregnancy (category C) or in nursing mothers is not established. Use with caution in the elderly.

Adverse/Side Effects: CNS: Drowsiness (usually transitory), sedation, dizziness, headache• CV: Chest tightness, hypotension• Respiratory: Dyspnea, wheezing• Skin: Injection site reactions, urticaria, erythematous macular eruptions• Other: Dry mouth, involuntary motor activity, erythema multiforme, phlebitis, hemolysis, thrombosis, digital gangrene from inadvertent IV or intra-arterial injection.

Interactions: Alcohol and CNS depressants add to CNS depression; tricyclic antidepressants and other anticholinergics have additive anticholinergic effects; may inhibit pressor effects of epinephrine.

Prehospital Considerations

- IM administration should be made deep into body of a relatively large muscle. The Z-track technique of injection is recommended to prevent SC infiltration.
- Recommended IM site: In adult, the gluteus maximus or vastus lateralis; in children, the vastus lateralis.
- Protect hydroxyzine from light. Store at 15–30C (59–86F) unless otherwise specified.
- Forewarn about the possibility of drowsiness and dizziness, and caution against hazardous activities until reaction to drug is known.
- Alcohol and hydroxyzine should not be taken at the same time.
- Care must be taken to NEVER give hydroxyzine intravenously.

IBUPROFEN

Class: Nonsteroidal anti-inflammatory drug (NSAID)

Trade Names: Actiprofen (Aus), Advil, Amersol (Can), Brufen (Aus), Children's Motrin, Excedrin IB, Genpril, Haltran, Ibuprin, Junior Strength Motrin Caplets, Medipren, Motrin, Nuprin, Nurofen (Aus), Pamprin-IB, Pediaprofen, Rafen (Aus), Rufen, Trendar

Therapeutic Action/Pharmacodynamics: Ibuprofen is the prototype NSAID with significant antipyretic and analgesic properties. It blocks prostaglandin synthesis, inhibits platelet aggregation, and prolongs bleeding time but does not affect prothrombin or whole blood clotting times. Cross-sensitivity with aspirin and other NSAIDs has been reported.

Emergency Uses: To reduce fever; to temporarily relieve mild to moderate pain. *Adult dose:* 200–400 mg PO every 4–6 hr up to 1,200 mg/day. *Pediatric dose:* 5–10 mg/kg PO every 4–6 hr up to 40 mg/kg/day.

Pharmacokinetics

Absorption: 80% absorbed from GI tract; onset is 1 hr. Antipyretic effect: peak is 1–2 hr; duration is 6–8 hr; half-life is 2–4 hr.
Metabolism: Metabolized in liver.
Elimination: Excreted primarily in urine; some biliary excretion.

Contraindications and Precautions: Ibuprofen is contraindicated in patients in whom urticaria, severe rhinitis, bronchospasm, angioedema, or nasal polyps are precipitated by aspirin or other NSAIDs; active peptic ulcer, bleeding abnormalities. Use with caution in patients with hypertension, history of GI ulceration, impaired hepatic or renal function, chronic renal failure, cardiac decompensation.

Adverse/Side Effects: CNS: Headache, dizziness, light-headedness, anxiety, emotional lability, fatigue, malaise, drowsiness, anxiety, confusion, depression, aseptic meningitis• CV: Hypertension, palpitations, congestive heart failure (patient with marginal cardiac function); peripheral edema• Eye/ear: Blurred vision, decreased visual acuity, changes in color vision, nystagmus, visual-field defects; tinnitus, impaired hearing• GI: Dry mouth, gingival ulcerations, dyspepsia, heartburn, nausea, vomiting, anorexia, diarrhea, constipation, bloating, flatulence, epigastric or abdominal discomfort or pain, GI ulceration, occult blood loss• Hematologic: Rise in bleeding time

• Renal: Acute renal failure, polyuria, azotemia, cystitis, hematuria, nephrotoxicity, decreased creatinine clearance
• Skin: Maculopapular and vesicobullous skin eruptions, erythema multiforme, pruritus, rectal itching, acne • Other: Fluid retention with edema, toxic hepatitis, hypersensitivity reactions, anaphylaxis, bronchospasm, angioedema.

Interactions: Ibuprofen may prolong bleeding time when used with anticoagulants. Also may increase lithium and methotrexate toxicity.

Prehospital Considerations
• Give on an empty stomach, 1 hr before or 2 hr after meals.
• If GI intolerance occurs, ibuprofen may be taken with meals or milk.
• Tablet may be crushed if patient is unable to swallow it whole and mixed with food or liquid before swallowing.
• Patients with history of cardiac decompensation should be observed closely for evidence of fluid retention and edema.
• Monitor for GI distress and signs of GI bleeding.
• Symptoms of acute toxicity in children are apnea, cyanosis, response only to painful stimuli, dizziness, and nystagmus.

Ibutilide

IBUTILIDE

Class: Antidysrhythmic

Trade Name: Corvert

Therapeutic Action/Pharmacodynamics: Ibutilide is a short-acting class III antidysrhythmic agent. It prolongs the cardiac action potential and increases both atrial and ventricular refractoriness (i.e., class III antidysrhythmic electrophysiologic effects). It is recommended for acute pharmacologic conversion of atrial flutter or atrial fibrillation or as an adjunct to electrical cardioversion in patients in whom electrical cardioversion alone has been ineffective. Its short duration of action makes it less effective than other antidysrhythmic agents for maintaining sinus rhythm once restored.

Emergency Uses: To convert atrial flutter or atrial fibrillation of relatively short duration. *Adult dose:* In patients weighing more than 60 kg, 1 mg over 10 min IV. In patients weighing less than 60 kg, 0.01 mg/kg IV. May repeat in 10 min if inadequate response.

Pharmacokinetics
Absorption: Onset is 30 min; half-life is 6 hr (range 2–21 hr).
Metabolism: Metabolized in liver.
Elimination: 82% excreted in urine, 19% in feces.

Contraindications and Precautions: Ibutilide is contraindicated in patients with a hypersensitivity to ibutilide, hypokalemia, and hypomagnesemia. Use with caution in patients with history of CHF, low ejection fraction, recent MI, prolonged QT intervals, liver disease, cardiovascular disorder other than atrial dysrhythmias, other drugs that prolong QT interval, lactation. Safety and effectiveness in children under 18 yr is not established.

Adverse/Side Effects: CNS: Headache • CV: Proarrhythmic effects (sustained and nonsustained polymorphic ventricular tachycardia), torsade de pointes, AV block, bundle branch block, ventricular extrasystoles, hypotension, postural hypotension, bradycardia, tachycardia, palpitations, prolonged QT segment • GI: Nausea.

Interactions: Increased potential for proarrhythmic effects when administered with astemizole, phenothiazines, tricyclic antidepressants, and terfenadine. Amiodarone, disopyramide, quinidine, procainamide, and sotalol may cause prolonged refractoriness if given within 4 hr of ibutilide.

Ibutilide

Prehospital Considerations

- IV preparation and administration: Contents of 1-mg vial may be given undiluted or diluted in 50 mL of 0.9% NaCl or D_5W to a concentration of 0.017 mg/mL. Infuse over 10 min.
- Stop IV infusion as soon as presenting dysrhythmia is terminated or with appearance of ventricular tachycardia or marked prolongation of QT or QTc.
- Class Ia and other class III antidysrhythmic drugs should not be given concurrently or within 4 hr of ibutilide.
- Observe with continuous ECG, BP, and HR monitoring during and for 4–6 hr after infusion or until QTc has returned to baseline. Monitor for longer periods with liver dysfunction or if prodysrhythmic activity is observed.
- Conversion to normal sinus rhythm normally occurs within 30 min of initiation of infusion.

INAMRINONE (formerly AMRINONE)

Classes: Cardiovascular agent; inotrope; vasodilator
Trade Name: Inocor
Therapeutic Action/Pharmacodynamics: A new chemical class of cardiac inotropic agents with vasodilator activity. Its mode of action appears to differ from that of the digitalis glycosides and beta-adrenergic stimulants. In patients with depressed myocardial function, it enhances myocardial contractility, increases cardiac output and stroke volume, and reduces right and left ventricular filling pressure, pulmonary capillary wedge pressure (PCWP), and systemic vascular resistance. It reduces afterload and preload by its direct relaxant effect on vascular smooth muscle. Inamrinone produces

hemodynamic improvements and symptomatic relief in patients in CHF due to ischemic heart disease.

Emergency Uses: For short-term management of CHF in patients not adequately controlled by traditional therapy, such as digitalis, diuretics, and vasodilators; may be used in conjunction with these agents. *Adult dose:* Loading dose of 0.75 mg/kg IV over 2–3 min, followed by maintenance infusion between 5 and 10 mcg/kg/min. *Pediatric dose:* Same as adult dosing formula.

Pharmacokinetics

Absorption: Onset is 2–5 min; peak effect in 10 min; duration is 2 hr; half-life is 3.6–7.5 hr.
Distribution: Unknown if it crosses placenta or into breast milk.
Metabolism: Metabolized in liver.
Elimination: Excreted primarily in urine.

Contraindications and Precautions: Hypersensitivity to inamrinone or to bisulfites; severe aortic or pulmonic valvular disease in lieu of appropriate surgery, acute MI; uncorrected hypokalemia or dehydration. Safe use during pregnancy (category C) and lactation or in children is not established. Use with caution in patients with compromised renal or hepatic function, arrhythmias, hypertrophic subaortic stenosis; decreased platelets. Concomitant cardiac glycoside therapy recommended in patients with atrial flutter or fibrillation.

Adverse/Side Effects: General: Hypersensitivity (pericarditis, pleuritis; myositis with interstitial shadows on chest x-ray and elevated sedimentation rate; vasculitis with nodular pulmonary densities, hypoxemia, ascites, jaundice) • CV: Hypotension, arrhythmias • Endocrine: Nephrogenic diabetes insipidus • GI: Nausea, vomiting, anorexia, abdominal cramps, hepatotoxicity • Hematologic: Asymptomatic thrombocytopenia.

Inamrinone

Interactions: Possibility of excessive hypotension with disopyramide.

Prehospital Considerations

- Monitor for therapeutic effectiveness: Increased cardiac output, decreased PCWP, relief of symptoms of CHF. Central venous pressure may be used to assess hypotension and blood volume.
- Monitor BP, heart rate, and respirations and keep physician informed. Rate of administration and duration of therapy are prescribed according to clinical response and adverse effects.
- In general, rate of infusion should be slowed or stopped with excessive drop in BP or arrhythmias.
- Monitor infusion site to prevent extravasation.
- Allergy alert: IV preparation contains sodium metabisulfite, a reducing agent to which certain susceptible individuals are allergic. Discontinue immediately if patient shows hypersensitivity reactions.
- Use infusion pump to regulate rate.

INSULIN

Class: Hormone

Trade Names: Actrapid (Aus), Humulin, Hypurin (Aus), Iletin, Novolin, Regular Insulin, Regular Purified Pork Insulin, Velosulin (Can)

Therapeutic Action/Pharmacodynamics: Insulin is a protein secreted by the beta cells of the islets of Langerhans in the pancreas. Insulin is responsible for promoting the uptake of glucose by the cells. When administered, it is distributed throughout the body. It combines with insulin receptors present on the cell membranes. This promotes glucose entry into the cell. In diabetics, where insulin secretion is diminished, supplemental insulin must be obtained by injection. Older forms of insulin are derived from animals (bovine and porcine). However, animal insulin is not identical to human insulin. Because of this, many patients will develop antibodies to animal insulin, rendering it less effective. Human insulin can be manufactured through genetic engineering (recombinant DNA technology). Genetically engineered insulin (Humulin, Novolin) is chemically identical to the insulin hormone secreted by the pancreas. Patients do not develop antibodies to human insulin as they do to animal insulin.

Emergency Uses: To reverse effects of hyperglycemia and diabetic coma. *Adult dose:* 5–10 U IV/IM/SC of regular insulin loading dose. Maintenance dose is based on blood glucose levels. *Pediatric dose:* 2–4 U IV/IM/SC of regular insulin loading dose. Maintenance dose is based on blood glucose levels.

Pharmacokinetics
Absorption: Rapidly absorbed from IM and SC injections. Onset is 0.5–1.0 hr; peak effect in 2–3 hr; duration is 5–7 hr; half-life is up to 13 hr.
Distribution: Throughout extracellular fluids.
Metabolism: Metabolized primarily in liver, with some metabolism in kidneys.
Elimination: Less than 2% excreted in urine.

Contraindications and Precautions: Seldom given in the prehospital setting. Contraindicated in patients with hypersensitivity to insulin animal protein and in hypoglycemia. Cautious use in pregnancy (category C).

Adverse/Side Effects: Hypersensitivity (usually occurs when insulin is at peak action point): Localized allergic reactions at injection site; generalized urticaria or bullae, lymphadenopathy, anaphylaxis (rare) • Hypoglycemia (hyperinsulinism): Profuse sweating, hunger, headache, nausea, tremulousness, tremors, palpitation, tachycardia, weakness, fatigue, nystagmus, circumoral pallor; numb mouth, tongue, and other paresthesias; visual disturbances (diplopia, blurred vision, mydriasis), staring expression, confusion, personality changes, ataxia, incoherent speech, apprehension, irritability, inability to concentrate, personality changes, uncontrolled yawning, loss of consciousness, delirium, hypothermia, convulsions, Babinski reflex, coma • Other: Posthypoglycemia or rebound hyperglycemia • Overdosage: psychic disturbances (i.e., aphasia, personality changes, maniacal behavior).

Interactions: Alcohol, anabolic steroids, MAO inhibitors, guanethidine, salicylates may potentiate hypoglycemic effects. Dextrothyroxine, corticosteroids, epinephrine may antagonize hypoglycemic effects. Furosemide, thiazide diuretics increase serum glucose levels. Propranolol and other beta blockers may mask symptoms of hypoglycemic reaction.

Prehospital Considerations
SC Administration
- Always use an insulin syringe.
- Regular insulin is generally administered 30 min before a meal.
- Avoid injection of cold insulin; it can lead to lipodystrophy, reduced rate of absorption, and local reactions.
- Commonly used injection sites are upper arms, thighs, abdomen (avoid area over urinary bladder and 2 in. [5 cm] around navel), buttocks, and upper back (if fat is loose enough to pick up).

IV Administration
- Regular insulin may be given by direct IV undiluted. Administer 10 U or a fraction thereof over 1 min. When insulin is administered by continuous infusion, rate must be ordered by physician.

- Regular insulin may be adsorbed into the container or tubing when added to an IV infusion solution. Amount lost is variable and depends on concentration of insulin, infusion system, contact duration, and flow rate. Monitor patient response closely.
- Insulin is stable at room temperature up to 1 month. Avoid exposure to direct sunlight or to temperature extremes (safe range is wide: 5–38C [40–100F]). Refrigerate but do not freeze stock supply. Insulin tolerates temperatures above 38C with less harm than freezing.
- Frequency of blood glucose monitoring is determined by the type of insulin regimen and health status of the patient.
- Monitor for hypoglycemia at time of peak action of insulin. Onset of hypoglycemia (blood sugar: 50–40 mg/dL) may be rapid and sudden.
- During treatment for ketoacidosis with IV insulin, check BP and blood glucose often.

IPECAC SYRUP

Class: Emetic

Trade Name: Syrup of Ipecac

Therapeutic Action/Pharmacodynamics: Ipecac is a potent and effective emetic used in the management of poisonings when vomiting is indicated. It acts as a local irritant on the gastric mucosa to induce vomiting and centrally on the chemoreceptor trigger zone (CTZ) in the medulla to induce vomiting.

Emergency Use: To induce vomiting of unabsorbed ingested poisons. *Adult dose:* 30 mL PO followed by 1–2 glasses of water; may repeat once in 20 min if necessary. *Pediatric dose:* 15 mL followed by 1–2 glasses of water; may repeat once in 20 min if necessary.

Pharmacokinetics
Absorption: Onset is 15–30 min; duration is 25 min.
Elimination: Metabolite can be detected in urine up to 60 days after excessive doses.

Contraindications and Precautions: Ipecac is contraindicated in any patient with an altered mental status or depressed gag reflex because of the risk of aspiration. Vomiting is also contraindicated in patients who have ingested caustic substances such as petroleum products, strong acids or alkalis, corrosives, and fast-acting CNS depressants. Avoid using ipecac when the ingested drug is an antiemetic, especially a phenothiazine. Because of the risk of aspiration associated with vomiting, the trend in the management of acute poisonings is to use activated charcoal.

Adverse/Side Effects: CNS: Convulsions, coma, sensory disturbances • CV: Cardiomyopathy, cardiotoxicity, cardiac dysrhythmias, atrial fibrillation, tachycardia, chest pain, hypotension, fatal myocarditis • Respiratory: Dyspnea • GI: Diarrhea, mild GI upset, vomiting, gastroenteritis, bloody diarrhea, stomach cramps, tremor.

Interactions: Do not administer syrup of ipecac with activated charcoal as the activated charcoal will nullify the effects of ipecac.

Prehospital Considerations
- Emetic effect occurs in 15–30 min and continues for 20–25 min. If vomiting does not occur in 20–30 min, the dose may be repeated once.
- If vomiting does not occur within 15–20 min after a second dose, contact physician immediately. Dosage should be recovered by gastric lavage and activated charcoal if necessary.
- The prehospital use of ipecac should be very limited to cases where the benefit of emesis outweighs the potential risks.

IPRATROPIUM

Class: Parasympatholytic bronchodilator
Trade Name: Atrovent
Therapeutic Action/Pharmacodynamics: Ipratroprium is an anticholinergic agent, chemically related to atropine. Given in a nebulized form, it acts directly on the smooth muscle of the bronchial tree by inhibiting acetylcholine at receptor sites. By blocking parasympathetic action, it dilates the bronchial smooth muscle and decreases secretions. It also abolishes the vagally mediated reflex bronchospasm caused by inhaled irritants such as smoke, dust, and cold air and by a range of inflammatory mediators (e.g., histamine).

Emergency Uses: To relieve bronchospasm in patients with reversible obstructive airway disease (asthma, chronic bronchitis, emphysema) and acute attacks of bronchospasm. *Adult dose:* 500 mcg in 2.5–3.0 mL via nebulizer or 2 inhalations from a metered dose inhaler (MDI). *Pediatric dose:* 125–250 mcg in 2.5–3.0 mL via nebulizer, or 1–2 inhalations from an MDI.

Pharmacokinetics
Absorption: 10% of inhaled dose reaches lower airway; approximately 0.5% of dose is systemically absorbed; peak effect in 1.5–2.0 hr; duration is 4–6 hr; half-life is 1.5–2 hr. *Elimination:* 48% of dose excreted in feces; less than 5% excreted in urine.

Contraindications and Precautions: Ipratroprium is contraindicated in patients with hypersensitivity to atropine or its derivatives. It should not be used as the primary treatment for acute episodes of bronchospasm. Cautious use in pregnancy (category B) and nursing mothers.

Adverse/Side Effects: Eye: Blurred vision (especially if sprayed into eye), difficulty in accommodation, acute eye pain, worsening of narrow-angle glaucoma • GI: Bitter taste, dry oropharyngeal membranes • With higher doses: Nausea, constipation • Respiratory: Cough, hoarseness, exacerbation of symptoms, drying of bronchial secretions, mucosal ulcers, epistaxis, nasal dryness • Other: Rash, hives, urinary retention, headache.

Prehospital Considerations

- Monitor respiratory status; auscultate lungs before and after inhalation.
- Treatment failure (exacerbation of respiratory symptoms) should be reported to physician.
- Ipratropium is almost always administered in conjunction with a beta-adrenergic agent such as albuterol.

ISOETHARINE

Class: Sympathomimetic bronchodilator

Trade Name: Bronkosol

Therapeutic Action/Pharmacodynamics: Isoetharine is a synthetic sympathomimetic stimulant with relatively rapid onset and long duration of action. The prime action of beta-adrenergic drugs is to stimulate adenyl cyclase, the enzyme that catalyzes the formation of cyclic-3,′ 5′-adenosine monophosphate (cyclic AMP) from adenosine triphosphate (ATP). The cyclic AMP causes relaxation of the smooth muscles of the bronchial tree, decreasing airway resistance, facilitating mucus drainage, and increasing vital capacity. It exerts minimal effects on $beta_1$ (heart) or alpha (peripheral vasculature) receptors. In therapeutic doses, isoetharine, by inhibiting histamine release from mast cells, also reduces the mucus secretion, capillary leaking, and mucosal edema caused by an allergic response in the lungs.

Emergency Uses: To relieve bronchospasm in patients with reversible obstructive airway disease (asthma, chronic bronchitis, emphysema) and acute attacks of bronchospasm. *Adult dose:* 1–2 inhalations via metered-dose inhaler; 0.5 mL of a 1% solution in 2–3 mL saline via nebulizer; 0.5 mL in 2–3 mL saline via bag-valve-mask (BVM). *Pediatric dose:* 0.01 mL/kg of 1% solution (maximum 0.5 mL) diluted in 2–3 mL normal saline.

Pharmacodynamics

Absorption: Onset is immediate; peak effect in 5–15 min; duration is 1–4 hr.

Metabolism: Metabolized in lungs, liver, GI tract, and other tissues.

Elimination: Excreted by kidneys.

Contraindications and Precautions: Isoetharine is contraindicated in patients with a known hypersensitivity to sympathomimetic amines and to bisulfites; concomitant use with epinephrine or other sympathomimetic amines; patients with preexisting cardiac dysrhythmias associated with tachycardia. Use with caution in elderly patients; hypertension; acute coronary artery disease; CHF; cardiac asthma; hyperthyroidism; diabetes mellitus; tuberculosis; history of seizures.

Adverse/Side Effects: CNS: Headache, anxiety, tension, restlessness, insomnia, tremor, weakness, dizziness, excitement • CV: Tachycardia, palpitations, changes in BP, cardiac arrest • GI: Nausea, vomiting • Respiratory: Cough, bronchial irritation, edema.

Interactions: Expect additive effects when used with epinephrine, other sympathomimetic bronchodilators. MAO inhibitors and tricyclic antidepressants may potentiate its action on the vascular system. If the patient is taking beta blockers, the effects of isoetharine will be antagonized.

Prehospital Considerations

- When using a metered-dose inhaler, instruct the patient to shake the container, exhale through nose as completely as possible, administer aerosol while inhaling deeply through mouth, and hold breath about 10 sec

Isoetharine

before exhaling slowly. Administer second inhalation 10 min after first.

- Monitor respiratory status. Measure peak flow and auscultate lungs before and after inhalation to determine efficacy of drug in decreasing airway resistance.
- Monitor cardiac status. Report tachycardia and hypotension.
- Drug may have shorter duration of action after long-term use. Instruct patient to report failure to respond to usual dose.
- Advise that tremor is an anticipated side effect.
- Isoetharine inhalation may be alternated with epinephrine or albuterol administration but may not be administered simultaneously because of danger of excessively rapid heartbeat.
- Do not use discolored or precipitated solutions.
- Elderly patients may be especially sensitive to adrenergic drug effects. Monitor cardiac status and report tachycardia and palpitations.
- Consider isoetharine for patients who have been extensively using another beta agonist such as albuterol. Because of tachyphylaxis, patients may experience decreased effectiveness of their usual beta agonist, and isoetharine may prove beneficial.

ISOPROTERENOL

Class: Sympathomimetic

Trade Name: Isuprel

Therapeutic Action/Pharmacodynamics: Isoproterenol is a synthetic sympathomimetic agonist with pure beta$_1$- and beta$_2$-adrenergic effects. Drug-induced stimulation of beta$_1$-adrenergic receptors results in increased cardiac output and work by increasing strength of cardiac contraction and, to a slight degree, rate of contraction. It produces a slight increase in systolic BP and decrease in diastolic pressure. Isoproterenol reduces total peripheral resistance and increases venous return to the heart by mobilizing blood from vascular reservoirs. Stimulation of beta$_2$-adrenoceptors relaxes bronchospasm and, by increasing ciliary motion, facilitates expectoration of pulmonary secretions. It also may dilate the trachea and main bronchi past the resting diameter.

Emergency Uses: To increase cardiac output by increasing the heart rate in symptomatic bradycardia refractory to atropine when transcutaneous pacing is not available. *Adult dose:* 2–10 mcg/min titrated to rate. *Pediatric dose:* 0.1 mcg/kg/min titrated to rate.

To dilate the bronchial tree in severe status asthmaticus. *Adult dose:* 1–2 inhalations of MDI. *Pediatric dose:* Same as for adult.

Pharmacokinetics
Absorption: Rapidly absorbed IV; immediate onset.
Metabolism: Action terminated by tissue uptake and metabolized by COMT in liver, lungs, and other tissues.
Elimination: 40–50% excreted in urine unchanged.

Contraindications and Precautions: Because isoproterenol increases preload, myocardial oxygen consumption, and demand, and reduces total peripheral resistance, it is contraindicated in patients in cardiogenic shock. Use with caution in patients with preexisting tachydysrhythmias associated with tachycardia, tachycardia caused by digitalis intoxication, and acute myocardial infarction.

Adverse/Side Effects: CNS: Headache, mild tremors, nervousness, anxiety, insomnia, excitement, fatigue • CV: Flushing, palpitations, tachycardia, unstable BP, anginal pain, ventricular dysrhythmias • Overdosage (especially

Isoproterenol

after excessive use of aerosols): Tachycardia, palpitations, nervousness, nausea, vomiting.

Interactions: Epinephrine and other sympathomimetic amines' effects are increased by isoproterenol and can potentially cause cardiac toxicity. Beta blockers antagonize these effects.

Prehospital Considerations
- IV infusion: Dilute 10 mL 1:5,000 solution in 500 mL 5% dextrose to produce a 1:250,000 solution.
- Microdrip or constant-infusion pump is recommended to prevent sudden influx of large amounts of drug.
- Infusion rate is generally decreased or infusion may be temporarily discontinued if heart rate exceeds 110 bpm, because of the danger of precipitating dysrhythmias.
- IV administration is regulated by continuous ECG monitoring. Patient must be observed, and response to therapy must be monitored continuously.
- Isoproterenol solutions lose potency with standing. Discard if precipitate or discoloration is present.
- Incidence of dysrhythmias is high, particularly when drug is administered IV to patients with cardiogenic shock or ischemic heart disease, to digitalized patients, or to those with electrolyte imbalance. Check pulse before and during IV administration. Rate greater than 110 usually indicates need to slow infusion rate or discontinue infusion. Consult physician for guidelines.
- Tolerance to bronchodilating effect and cardiac stimulant effect may develop with prolonged use.
- Rebound bronchospasm may occur when effects of drug end. Once tolerance has developed, continued use can result in serious adverse effects.
- With the advent of transcutaneous pacing, isoproterenol has a very minimal role in modern prehospital care.

KETOROLAC

Class: Nonsteroidal anti-inflammatory drug (NSAID)

Trade Names: Toradol

Therapeutic Action/Pharmacodynamics: Ketorolac is an injectable NSAID that exhibits analgesic, anti-inflammatory, and antipyretic activity. It works by inhibiting the synthesis of prostaglandins. Ketorolac does not have any known effects on opiate receptors. Unlike narcotics, which act on the central nervous system, ketorolac does not have the sedative properties and is a peripherally acting analgesic. It is the first injectable NSAID to become available in the United States.

Emergency Use: To relieve mild to moderate pain. *Adult dose:* IV loading dose: 30 mg (15 mg if patient is older than 65 yr or weighs less than 50 kg). IM: 30–60 mg loading dose. *Pediatric dose:* Rarely used.

Pharmacokinetics
Absorption: Peak effects in 45–60 min; half-life is 4–6 hr.
Distribution: Distributed into breast milk.
Metabolism: Metabolized in liver.
Elimination: Excreted in urine.

Contraindications and Precautions: Ketorolac is contraindicated in patients with asthma and with hypersensitivity to ketorolac, aspirin, or other NSAIDs. Use with caution in patients with a history of peptic ulcers; impaired renal or hepatic function; elderly.

Adverse/Side Effects: CNS: Drowsiness, dizziness, headache • GI: Nausea, dyspepsia, GI pain, hemorrhage • Other: Edema, sweating, pain at injection site.

Interactions: Ketorolac may increase lithium levels and toxicity. It also may worsen the side effects of aspirin and other NSAIDs when used in conjunction with them. Ketorolac has been found to reduce the diuretic response to furosemide.

Prehospital Considerations

- When used for pain relief, reduced dosages may be necessary with the elderly because of renal effects of NSAIDs.
- Inject IM ketorolac slowly and deeply into a large muscle.
- Injection site pain has been reported in some patients receiving multiple doses. Rotate injection sites.
- Administer IV bolus dose over at least 15 sec.
- Hypovolemia should be corrected prior to administration of ketorolac.
- Monitor for signs and symptoms of bleeding. Ketorolac decreases platelet aggregation and thus may prolong bleeding time.
- Monitor for signs and symptoms of GI distress or bleeding, including nausea, GI pain, diarrhea, melena, or hematemesis. GI ulceration with perforation can occur anytime during treatment.
- Patients with a history of cardiac decompensation should be observed closely for evidence of fluid retention and edema.
- When administering ketorolac intravenously, always use a dose of 30 mg or less. The IM dose is 30–60 mg.

LABETALOL

Class: Beta blocker

Trade Names: Normodyne, Presolol (Aus), Trandate

Therapeutic Action/Pharmacodynamics: Labetalol is an adrenergic-receptor blocking agent that combines selective alpha activity and nonselective beta-adrenergic blocking actions. Both activities contribute to reduce blood pressure. Alpha blockade results in vasodilation, decreased peripheral resistance, and orthostatic hypotension and only slightly affects cardiac output and coronary artery blood flow. Beta-blocking effects on sinus node, AV node, and ventricular muscle lead to bradycardia, delay in AV conduction, and depression of cardiac contractility.

Emergency Use: To manage an acute hypertensive crisis. *Adult dose:* 20 mg slow IV with 40–80 mg every 10 min as needed up to 300 mg total, or 2 mg/min continuous infusion up to 300 mg total dose. *Pediatric dose:* Safety in children has not been established.

Pharmacokinetics
Absorption: Onset is 2–5 min IV; peak effects in 5–15 min; duration is 2–4 hr; half-life is 3–8 hr.
Distribution: Crosses placenta; distributed into breast milk.
Metabolism: Metabolized in liver.
Elimination: 60% excreted in urine, 40% in bile.

Contraindications and Precautions: Because it is a nonselective beta blocker, labetalol is contraindicated in bronchial asthma. It is also contraindicated in uncontrolled cardiac failure, heart block (greater than first degree), cardiogenic shock, and severe bradycardia. Safe use during pregnancy (category C), in nursing women, and in children is not established. Use with caution in patients with nonallergic bronchospastic disease (COPD), well-compensated patients with history of heart failure; pheochromocytoma; impaired hepatic function, jaundice; diabetes mellitus; peripheral vascular disease.

Adverse/Side Effects: CNS: Dizziness, fatigue/malaise, headache, tremors, transient paresthesias (especially scalp tingling), hypoesthesia (numbness), mental depression, drowsiness, sleep disturbances, nightmares • CV: Postural hypotension, angina pectoris, palpitation, bradycardia, syncope, pedal or peripheral edema, pulmonary edema, CHF, flushing, cold extremities, dysrhythmias (following IV), paradoxical hypertension (patients with pheochromocytoma) • Eye: Dry eyes, vision disturbances • GI: Nausea, vomiting, dyspepsia, constipation, diarrhea, taste disturbances, cholestasis with or without jaundice, increases in serum transaminases, dry mouth • GU: Acute urinary retention, difficult micturition, impotence, ejaculation failure, loss of libido • Respiratory: Dyspnea, bronchospasm • Skin: Rashes of various types, increased sweating, pruritus • Other: Nasal stuffiness, rhinorrhea, myalgia, muscle cramps, pain at IV injection site.

Interactions: Cimetidine may increase the effects of labetalol; beta agonists antagonize effects of labetalol. Other antihypertensive agents may potentiate the effects of labetalol. Do not use with IV calcium channel blockers.

Prehospital Considerations

- Patient should be supine when receiving labetalol IV due to orthostatic hypotension. Take BP immediately before administration.
- Drug may be given undiluted by direct IV or further diluted in most IV solutions and administered as a continuous infusion.
- Continuous IV infusion: Rate is adjusted according to BP response. Normal rate is 2 mg/min. Once the desired BP is attained, labetalol is discontinued.
- Controlled-infusion pump device is recommended for maintaining accurate flow rate during IV infusion. Usually administered at rate of 2 mg/min.
- Monitor BP and pulse during dosage adjustment period. Standing BP is used often as an indicator for making dosage adjustments and for assessing patient's tolerance of dosage increases. Generally taken after patient stands for 10 min. Clarify with physician.
- After IV administration, (1) monitor BP at 5-min intervals for 30 min; (2) then at 30-min intervals for 2 hr; (3) then hourly for about 6 hr, and as indicated thereafter.
- Supine position should be maintained for at least 3 hr after IV administration. At the end of this time, determine

patient's ability to tolerate elevated and upright positions before allowing ambulation. Manage this slowly.

- Instruct patient to make all position changes slowly and in stages, particularly from recumbent to upright position. Elderly patients are especially sensitive to hypotensive effects.
- Since labetalol can cause dizziness and light-headedness, advise to avoid potentially hazardous activities until reaction to drug is known.
- Diabetic patients should be closely monitored. Labetalol may mask usual cardiovascular response to acute hypoglycemia, e.g., tachycardia.
- Reassure patient that most adverse effects (e.g., scalp tingling) are mild, transient, and dose related and occur early in therapy.

LEVALBUTEROL

Class: Sympathomimetic bronchodilator

Trade Name: Xopenex

Therapeutic Action/Pharmacodynamics: Levalbuterol acts on the beta$_2$ receptors of the smooth muscles of the bronchial tree, thus resulting in bronchodilation. It decreases airway resistance, facilitates mucus drainage, and increases vital capacity.

Emergency Uses: Treatment or prevention of bronchospasm in patients with reversible obstructive airway disease. *Adult dose:* 0.63 mcg by nebulizer. *Pediatric dose:* 6–11 yr: 0.31 mcg by nebulizer; over 11 yr follow adult dosing scheme.

Pharmacokinetics

Absorption: Onset in 5–15 min; duration is of 3–6 hr; half-life is 3.3 hr.

Contraindications and Precautions: Hypersensitivity to levalbuterol or albuterol; angioedema; pregnancy (category C); children under 6 yr; lactation. Use with caution in patients with cardiovascular disorders, especially coronary insufficiency, cardiac arrhythmias, hypertension, QT elongation, convulsive disorders; diabetes mellitus, diabetic ketoacidosis; older adults; seizures, status asthmaticus, tachycardia; hypersensitivity to sympathetic amines; hyperthyroidism, thyrotoxicosis.

Adverse/Side Effects: General: Allergic reactions, flu syndrome, pain • CNS: Migraine, dizziness, nervousness, tremor, anxiety • CV: Tachycardia • GI: Dyspepsia • Respiratory: Increased cough, viral infection, rhinitis, sinusitis, turbinate edema, paradoxical bronchospasm • Endocrine: Increase in serum glucose.

Interactions: Beta blockers may antagonize levalbuterol effects; MAO inhibitors and tricyclic antidepressants may potentiate levalbuterol effects on vascular system; ECG changes or hypokalemia may be exacerbated by loop or thiazide diuretics.

Prehospital Considerations
- Use vials within 2 wk of opening pouch. Protect vial from light and use within 1 wk after removal from pouch. Use only if solution in vial is colorless.
- Monitor for signs and symptoms of CNS or cardiovascular stimulation (e.g., BP, HR, respiratory status).

LIDOCAINE

Class: Antidysrhythmic

Trade Names: Xylocaine, Xylocard (Aus, Can)

Therapeutic Action/Pharmacodynamics: Lidocaine has cardiac actions similar to those of procainamide and quinidine but has little effect on myocardial contractility, AV and intraventricular conduction, cardiac output, and systolic arterial pressure in equivalent doses. It exerts antidysrhythmic action (class Ib) by suppressing automaticity in the His-Purkinje system and by elevating electrical stimulation threshold of ventricle during diastole. It is used to raise the threshold for ventricular dysrhythmias and to lower the threshold for defibrillation and cardioversion. Progressive depression of CNS occurs with increasing blood concentration; produces anticonvulsant, sedative, and analgesic effects.

Emergency Uses: To convert ventricular dysrhythmias (ventricular fibrillation, ventricular tachycardia) in cardiac arrest to sinus rhythm. *Adult dose:* 1.0–1.5 mg/kg IV. Repeat every 3–5 min as needed up to 3 mg/kg. Following conversion, begin infusion at 2–4 mg/min. *Pediatric dose:* 1 mg/kg IV. Repeat as needed every 3–5 min up to 3 mg/kg. Following conversion, begin infusion at 20–50 mcg/kg/min.

To convert ventricular tachycardia with a pulse to sinus rhythm. *Adult dose:* 1.0–1.5 mg/kg slow IV. May repeat at one-half dose every 5–10 min until conversion up to 3 mg/kg. Following conversion, begin infusion at 2–4 mg/min. *Pediatric dose:* 1 mg/kg IV followed by an infusion at 20–50 mcg/kg/min.

Pharmacokinetics
Absorption: Onset in under 3 min; peak effects in 5–7 min; duration is 10–20 min; half-life is 1.5–2.0 hr.
Distribution: Crosses blood-brain barrier and placenta; distributed into breast milk.
Metabolism: Metabolized in liver.
Elimination: Excreted in urine.

Contraindications and Precautions: Lidocaine is contraindicated in patients with a history of hypersensitivity to amide-type local anesthetics, supraventricular dysrhythmias, Stokes-Adams syndrome, untreated sinus bradycardia, severe degrees of sinoatrial, atrioventricular, and intraventricular heart block. Use with caution in patients with liver or renal disease, CHF, marked hypoxia, respiratory depression, hypovolemia, shock; myasthenia gravis; debilitated patients, the elderly; family history of malignant hyperthermia (fulminant hypermetabolism).

Adverse/Side Effects: CNS: Drowsiness, dizziness, light-headedness, restlessness, confusion, disorientation, irritability, apprehension, euphoria, wild excitement, numbness of lips or tongue, and other paresthesias, including sensations of heat and cold, chest heaviness, difficulty in speaking, difficulty in breathing or swallowing, muscular twitching, tremors, psychosis • With high doses: Convulsions, respiratory depression and arrest • CV: (with high doses): Hypotension, bradycardia, conduction disorders, including heart block, cardiovascular collapse, cardiac arrest • Ears: Tinnitus, decreased hearing • Eye: Blurred or double vision, impaired color perception • Other: Anorexia, nausea, vomiting, excessive perspiration, soreness at IV site, local thrombophlebitis (with prolonged IV infusion), hypersensitivity reactions (urticaria, rash, edema, anaphylactoid reactions).

Interactions: Barbiturates decrease lidocaine activity. Cimetidine, beta blockers, and quinidine increase the pharmacologic effects of lidocaine. Phenytoin increases its cardiac depressant effects; procainamide compounds neurologic and cardiac effects.

Prehospital Considerations
- Only lidocaine hydrochloride injection without preservatives that is specifically labeled for IV use should be used for IV injection or infusion.
- Bolus dose of lidocaine may be given undiluted by direct IV at a rate of 50 mg or fraction thereof over 1 min.
- Lidocaine may be added to D_5W or NS for infusion. For adults, add 1 g to 250–500 mL; for children, add 120 mg to 100 mL.

- For IV infusion, use microdrop tubing and infusion pump. Rate of flow is usually no more than 4 mg/min.
- IV infusion should be terminated as soon as patient's basic cardiac rhythm stabilizes or at earliest signs and symptoms of toxicity (infusions are rarely continued beyond 24 hr).
- Inspect solutions for particulate matter and discoloration prior to administration and discard if either is present.
- If ECG signs of excessive cardiac depression occur, such as prolongation of PR interval or QRS complex and the appearance or aggravation of dysrhythmias, infusion should be stopped immediately.
- Constant ECG monitoring and frequent determinations of BP, respirations, and CNS status are essential to avoid potential overdosage and toxicity.
- Auscultate lungs for basilar rales, especially in patients who tend to metabolize the drug slowly (e.g., CHF, cardiogenic shock, hepatic dysfunction).
- In patients receiving IV infusions of lidocaine or those with high lidocaine blood levels, watch for neurotoxic effects: drowsiness, dizziness, confusion, paresthesias, visual disturbances, excitement, dysarthria, behavioral changes.
- The role of lidocaine in advanced life support is more limited based on recent AHA guidelines. Prophylactic lidocaine should not be used. Lidocaine is now considered second-line therapy behind amiodarone, procainamide, and sotalol.

LORAZEPAM

Class: Sedative

Trade Names: Apo-Lorazepam (Aus), Ativan, Novo-Lorazepam, Nu-Loraz (Can)

Therapeutic Action/Pharmacodynamics: Lorazepam is the most potent of the available benzodiazepines. Its effects (anxiolytic, sedative, hypnotic, and skeletal muscle relaxant) are mediated by the inhibitory neurotransmitter GABA. Action sites include the thalamic, hypothalamic, and limbic levels of CNS. Lorazepam has a shorter half-life than diazepam and is used as a premedication for cardioversion and minor surgery because it induces amnesia and reduces the patient's recall of the procedure. Like diazepam, it suppresses the spread of seizure activity through the motor cortex of the brain while not abolishing the abnormal discharge focus. Because of its short half-life, it is a preferred drug for pediatric seizures. Unlike diazepam (Valium), lorazepam is water soluble and can be easily diluted for administration.

Emergency Uses: To induce sedation for cardioversion. *Adult dose:* 2–4 mg IM; 0.5–2 mg IV. *Pediatric dose:* 0.03–0.05 mg/kg IV/IM/PR up to 4 mg.

To manage status epilepticus. *Adult dose:* 2 mg slow IV (2 mg/min). *Pediatric dose:* 0.1 mg/kg slow IV (over 2–5 min); repeat one-half dose as needed. The drug may be given rectally if an IV cannot be placed.

Pharmacokinetics

Absorption: Onset is 1–5 min IV, 15–30 min IM; peak effects in 15–20 min IV, 2 hr IM; duration is 6–8 hr; half-life is 10–20 hr.
Distribution: Crosses placenta; distributed into breast milk.
Metabolism: Metabolized in liver.
Elimination: Excreted in urine.

Contraindications and Precautions: Lorazepam is contraindicated in patients with known sensitivity to benzodiazepines, children younger than 12 yr (PO preparation), pregnancy (category D), and nursing mothers. Use with caution in patients with acute narrow-angle glaucoma; primary depressive disorders or psychosis; coma, shock, acute alcohol intoxication, renal or hepatic impairment; organic brain syndrome; myasthenia gravis; narrow-angle glaucoma; suicidal tendency; GI disorders; elderly and debilitated patients; limited pulmonary reserve.

Adverse/Side Effects: CNS: Anterograde amnesia, drowsiness, sedation, dizziness, weakness, unsteadiness, disorientation, depression, sleep disturbance, restlessness, confusion, hallucinations• CV: Hypertension or hypotension• Eye: Blurred vision, diplopia• Ear: Depressed hearing• GI: Nausea, vomiting, abdominal discomfort, anorexia.

Interactions: Alcohol, CNS depressants, and anticonvulsants may potentiate CNS depression. Cimetidine increases lorazepam plasma levels and increases toxicity. Lorazepam may decrease antiparkinsonism effects of levodopa; may increase phenytoin levels; smoking decreases its sedative and antianxiety effects.

Prehospital Considerations

- IM lorazepam is injected undiluted, deep into a large muscle mass.
- IV preparation: Prepare lorazepam immediately before use. Dilute with an equal volume of sterile water, D_5W, or NS. Do not use a discolored solution or one that has a precipitate.
- IV administration: Diluted drug is injected directly into vein or into IV infusion tubing at rate not to exceed 2 mg/min and with repeated aspiration to confirm IV entry.
- IV administration to neonates, infants, children: Verify correct IV concentration and rate of infusion with physician.
- Flumazenil, a benzodiazepine antagonist, should be available.
- Extreme precautions should be taken to prevent intra-arterial injection and perivascular extravasation.

- Patients older than 50 yr may have more profound and prolonged sedation with IV lorazepam. Usually, an initial dose of 2 mg should not be exceeded.
- Keep parenteral preparation in refrigerator; do not freeze. Store tablets at 15–30C (59–86F) unless manufacturer specifies otherwise.
- Equipment for maintaining patent airway should be immediately available before IV administration.
- IM or IV lorazepam injection of 2–4 mg is usually followed by a depth of drowsiness or sleepiness that permits patient to respond to simple instructions whether patient appears to be asleep or awake.

MAGNESIUM SULFATE

Class: Electrolyte

Trade Name: Magnesium

Therapeutic Action/Pharmacodynamics: Magnesium sulfate is an essential element in many biochemical processes that occur within the body. It acts as a physiologic calcium channel blocker and blocks neuromuscular transmission. Hypomagnesemia (decreased magnesium levels) can cause cardiac dysrhythmias, including refractory ventricular fibrillation. It also can result in symptoms of cardiac insufficiency and sudden cardiac death. When given parenterally, it acts as a CNS depressant and also a depressant of smooth, skeletal, and cardiac muscle function. It has anticonvulsant properties thought to be produced by CNS depression, principally by decreasing the amount of acetylcholine liberated from motor nerve terminals, thus producing peripheral neuromuscular blockade.

Emergency Uses: To reverse refractory ventricular fibrillation and pulseless ventricular tachycardia (especially torsade). *Adult dose:* 1–2 g IV over 1–2 min. *Pediatric dose:* 25–50 mg/kg IV/IM.

To reverse torsades de pointes. *Adult dose:* 1–2 g IV followed by infusion of 0.5–1.0 g/hr IV. *Pediatric dose:* 25–50 mg/kg IV/IM.

To provide prophylaxis following acute myocardial infarction. *Adult dose:* 1–2 g IV over 5–30 min. *Pediatric dose:* Not used.

To manage seizures caused by eclampsia. *Adult dose:* 2–4 g IV/IM. *Pediatric dose:* Not used.

Pharmacokinetics

Absorption: Onset is immediate IV, 1 hr IM; duration is 30 min.

Distribution: Crosses placenta; distributed into breast milk.

Elimination: Eliminated in kidneys.

Contraindications and Precautions: Magnesium is contraindicated in patients with myocardial damage, heart block, shock, persistent hypertension, hypocalcemia. Use with caution in patients with impaired renal function, digitalized patients, concomitant use of other CNS depressants or neuromuscular blocking agents.

Adverse/Side Effects: CNS: Sedation, confusion, depressed reflexes or no reflexes, muscle weakness, flaccid paralysis • CV: Hypotension, depressed cardiac function, complete heart block, circulatory collapse • Respiratory: Respiratory paralysis • Other: Flushing, sweating, extreme thirst, hypothermia, respiratory paralysis, hypocalcemia.

Interactions: Neuromuscular blocking agents add to respiratory depression and apnea. If administered in conjunction with digitalis, cardiac conduction abnormalities can occur.

Magnesium Sulfate

Prehospital Considerations

- Administer magnesium slowly to minimize side effects.
- IV administration to infants, children: Verify correct IV concentration and rate of infusion with physician.
- When magnesium sulfate is given IV, patient requires constant observation. Check BP and pulse every 10–15 min or more often if indicated.
- Early indicators of magnesium toxicity (hypermagnesemia) include cathartic effect, profound thirst, feeling of warmth, sedation, confusion, depressed deep tendon reflexes, and muscle weakness.
- Before each repeated parenteral dose, patellar reflex should be tested. Depression or absence of reflexes is a useful index of early magnesium intoxication.
- Calcium chloride or calcium gluconate should be available as an antidote if serious side effects occur.
- Newborns of mothers who received parenteral magnesium sulfate within a few hours of delivery should be observed for signs of toxicity, including respiratory and neuromuscular depression.
- The role of magnesium sulfate in the management of refractory bronchospasm remains controversial. Consult with your medical director regarding use of magnesium sulfate in such conditions.

MANNITOL

Class: Osmotic diuretic

Trade Name: Osmitrol

Therapeutic Action/Pharmacodynamics: Mannitol is an osmotic diuretic that, through its hypertonic effects, draws water into the intravascular space. Then it induces diuresis by raising osmotic pressure of glomerular filtrate, thereby inhibiting tubular reabsorption of water and solutes. It is an effective way to reduce intracranial pressure and cerebral edema. In large doses, it may increase rate of electrolyte excretion, particularly sodium, chloride, and potassium. Mannitol reduces elevated intraocular and cerebrospinal pressures by increasing plasma osmolality, thus inducing diffusion of water from these fluids back into plasma and extravascular space.

Emergency Use: To reduce acute cerebral edema. *Adult dose:* 1.5–2.0 g/kg slow IV infusion. *Pediatric dose:* 0.25–0.5 g/kg IV over 60 min.

Pharmacokinetics

Absorption: Onset is 15 min; duration is 3–8 hr; half-life is 100 min.
Distribution: Confined to extracellular space; does not cross blood-brain barrier except with very high plasma levels in the presence of acidosis.
Metabolism: Small quantity metabolized to glycogen in liver.
Elimination: Rapidly excreted by kidneys.

Contraindications and Precautions: Mannitol is contraindicated in patients with marked pulmonary edema or CHF, organic CNS disease, intracranial bleeding; shock, severe dehydration, or history of allergy; pregnancy (category C).

Adverse/Side Effects: CNS: Headache, tremor, convulsions, dizziness, transient muscle rigidity • CV: Edema, CHF, angina-like pain, hypotension, hypertension, thrombophlebitis • Eye: Blurred vision • GI: Dry mouth, nausea, vomiting • GU: Marked diuresis, urinary retention, nephrosis, uricosuria • Metabolic: Fluid and electrolyte imbalance, especially hyponatremia; dehydration, acidosis • Other: With extravasation: local edema, skin necrosis; chills, fever, allergic reactions.

Interactions: Mannitol should not be administered with whole blood or packed red cells as it can damage the red blood cells.

Mannitol

Prehospital Considerations

- Concentrations higher than 15% have a greater tendency to crystallize. Administration set with an in-line IV filter should be used when infusing concentrations of 15% or above.
- Store preferably at 15–30C (59–86F) unless otherwise directed. Avoid freezing. If mannitol does crystallize, warm it slowly in boiling water until the crystals disappear.
- Care should be taken to avoid extravasation. Observe injection site for signs of inflammation or edema.
- Monitor vital signs and carefully note possible indications of fluid and electrolyte imbalance (e.g., thirst, muscle cramps or weakness, paresthesias, and signs of CHF).
- Be alert to the possibility that a rebound increase in ICP sometimes occurs about 12 hr after drug administration. Patient may complain of headache or confusion.

MEPERIDINE

Class: Narcotic analgesic

Trade Name: Demerol

Therapeutic Action/Pharmacodynamics: Meperidine is a synthetic narcotic central nervous system depressant with analgesic and sedative properties comparable to morphine, but without the hemodynamic effects. Meperidine is chemically dissimilar to morphine, yet it has the same tendency for physical dependency and abuse as morphine. Also, unlike morphine, it has little or no antidiarrheic or antitussive action and produces CNS stimulation in toxic doses. Its rate of onset is slightly faster than that of morphine, yet its effects are much shorter in duration.

Usual doses produce either no pupillary change or slight miosis, but overdosage results in marked miosis or mydriasis.

Emergency Use: To relieve moderate to severe pain. *Adult dose:* 25–50 mg IV; 50–100 mg IM. *Pediatric dose:* 1 mg/kg IV/IM.

Pharmacokinetics

Absorption: Onset is 5 min IV, 10 min IM; peak effect in 1 hour; duration is 2 hr IV, 2–4 hr IM; half-life is 3–5 hr.
Distribution: Crosses placenta; distributed into breast milk.
Metabolism: Metabolized in liver.
Elimination: Excreted in urine.

Contraindications and Precautions: Meperidine is contraindicated in patients with hypersensitivity to meperidine, convulsive disorders, acute abdominal conditions prior to diagnosis. Use with caution in patients with head injuries, increased intracranial pressure, asthma and other respiratory conditions, supraventricular tachycardias, prostatic hypertrophy, urethral stricture, glaucoma, elderly or debilitated patients, impaired renal or hepatic function, hypothyroidism, Addison's disease.

Adverse/Side Effects: Allergic: Pruritus, urticaria, skin rashes, wheal and flare over IV site • CNS: Dizziness, weakness, euphoria, dysphoria, sedation, headache, uncoordinated muscle movements, disorientation, decreased cough reflex, miosis, corneal anesthesia, respiratory depression. Toxic doses: muscle twitching, tremors, hyperactive reflexes, excitement, hypersensitivity to external stimuli, agitation, confusion, hallucinations, dilated pupils, convulsions • CV: Facial flushing, light-headedness, hypotension, syncope, palpitation, bradycardia, tachycardia, cardiovascular collapse, cardiac arrest (toxic doses) • GI: Dry mouth, nausea, vomiting, constipation, biliary tract spasm • Other: Oliguria, urinary retention, profuse perspiration, respiratory depression in newborn, bronchoconstriction (large doses), phlebitis (following IV use), pain, tissue irritation and induration.

Interactions: Alcohol and other CNS depressants and cimetidine cause additive sedation and CNS depression. Amphetamines may potentiate CNS stimulation. MAO inhibitors, selegiline, and furazolidone may cause excessive and prolonged CNS depression, convulsions, cardiovascular collapse. Phenytoin may increase toxic meperidine metabolites.

Prehospital Considerations

- Meperidine may cause respiratory depression. Have naloxone available as an antidote.
- Meperidine is a Schedule II controlled substance. Always keep secured in a locked box.
- Carefully aspirate before giving IM injection to avoid inadvertent IV administration. IV injection of undiluted drug can cause a marked increase in heart rate and syncope.
- IV injection: When meperidine is given by direct IV, dilute 50 mg in a minimum of 5 mL of NS or sterile water to yield 10 mg/mL. Inject it slowly at a rate not to exceed 25 mg/min. Slower injection preferred.
- IV infusion: When meperidine is given by continuous infusion, dilute it to a concentration of 1–10 mg/mL in NS, D_5W, or other compatible solution. Infusion rate should not exceed 25 mg/min. Slower rate is preferred.
- IV administration to infants, children: Verify correct IV concentration and rate of infusion/injection with physician.
- Narcotic analgesics should be given in the smallest effective dose and for the least period of time compatible with patient's needs.

- In patients receiving repeated doses, note respiratory rate, depth, and rhythm, and size of pupils. If respirations are 12/min or below and pupils are constricted or dilated (see actions and uses) or breathing is shallow, or if signs of CNS hyperactivity are present, consult physician before administering drug.
- Vital signs should be monitored closely. Heart rate may increase markedly, and hypotension may occur. Meperidine may cause severe hypotension in postoperative patients and those with depleted blood volume.
- Deep breathing, coughing (unless contraindicated), and changes in position at scheduled intervals may help to overcome the respiratory depressant effects of meperidine.
- Parenteral administration has caused corneal anesthesia and thus abolishment of corneal reflex in some patients. Be alert for this possibility.
- Monitor the patient's response to meperidine and report any changes to medical control.

METAPROTERENOL

Class: Sympathomimetic bronchodilator

Trade Names: Alupent, Metaprel

Therapeutic Action/Pharmacodynamics: Potent synthetic sympathomimetic amine similar to isoproterenol in chemical structure and pharmacologic actions. Metaproterenol is a relatively selective beta$_2$-adrenergic. The prime action of beta-adrenergic drugs is to stimulate adenyl cyclase, the enzyme that catalyzes the formation of cyclic-3′, 5′-adenosine monophosphate (cyclic AMP) from adenosine triphosphate (ATP). The cyclic AMP causes relaxation of the smooth muscles of the bronchial tree, decreasing airway resistance, facilitating mucus drainage, and increasing vital capacity. It exerts minimal effects on beta$_1$ (heart) or alpha (peripheral vasculature) receptors. In therapeutic doses, metaproterenol, by inhibiting histamine release from mast cells, also reduces the mucus secretion, capillary leaking, and mucosal edema caused by an allergic response in the lungs.

Emergency Use: To relieve bronchospasm in patients with reversible obstructive airway disease (asthma, chronic bronchitis, emphysema) and acute attacks of bronchospasm. *Adult dose:* 0.65 mg via metered-dose inhaler (2 sprays); 0.2–0.3 mL in 2.5–3.0 mL saline via nebulizer. *Pediatric dose:* 0.1–0.2 mL/kg of 5% solution in 2.5–3.0 mL saline via nebulizer.

Pharmacokinetics
Absorption: Onset is 1 min; peak effect in 1 hr; duration is 1–5 hr.
Metabolism: Metabolized in liver.
Elimination: Excreted in urine.

Contraindications and Precautions: Metaproterenol is contraindicated in patients with sensitivity to other sympathomimetic agents; cardiac dysrhythmias associated with tachycardia; and hyperthyroidism. Use with caution in the elderly and those with hypertension, coronary artery disease, and diabetes.

Adverse/Side Effects: CNS: Nervousness, weakness, drowsiness, tremor, headache, fatigue • CV: Tachycardia, hypertension, cardiac arrest, palpitation • GI: Nausea, vomiting, bad taste • Other: Occasional difficulty in micturition and muscle cramps, throat irritation, cough, exacerbation of asthma.

Interactions: Expect additive effects when used with epinephrine, other sympathomimetic bronchodilators. MAO inhibitors and tricyclic antidepressants may potentiate its action on the vascular system. If your patient is taking beta blockers, the effects of metaproterenol will be antagonized.

Prehospital Considerations

- When using a metered-dose inhaler, instruct the patient to shake the container, exhale through nose as completely as possible, administer aerosol while inhaling deeply through mouth, and hold breath about 10 sec before exhaling slowly. Administer second inhalation 10 min after first.
- Monitor respiratory status. Measure peak flow and auscultate lungs before and after inhalation to determine efficacy of drug in decreasing airway resistance.
- Monitor cardiac status. Report tachycardia and hypotension.
- Advise that tremor is an anticipated side effect.
- Do not use discolored or precipitated solutions.
- Elderly patients may be especially sensitive to adrenergic drug effects. Monitor cardiac status and report tachycardia and palpitations.

METARAMINOL

Class: Sympathomimetic

Trade Name: Aramine

Therapeutic Action/Pharmacodynamics: Metaraminol is a potent synthetic sympathomimetic agonist. Its overall effects are similar to those of norepinephrine, but it is not as potent, has more gradual onset and longer duration of action, and usually lacks CNS stimulant effects. Metaraminol acts directly on alpha-adrenergic receptors (vasoconstriction) and also directly stimulates $beta_1$ receptors of heart (positive inotropic effect); indirectly causes release of norepinephrine from storage sites.

Its vasoconstrictor action increases pulmonary arterial pressure, produces sustained rise in systolic and diastolic pressures, and reduces blood flow to the kidneys. Once used to raise blood pressure in low-flow states, it is rarely used today because dopamine has become the preferred agent.

Emergency Use: To manage hemodynamically significant hypotension not due to hypovolemia. *Adult dose:* 100 mg in 500 mL of D_5W or NS titrated to BP response; 5–10 mg IM. *Pediatric dose:* Not used.

Pharmacokinetics
Absorption: Onset is 1–2 min IV, <10 min IM; duration is 20–90 min.
Metabolism: Metabolized in tissues.
Elimination: Excreted in urine.

Contraindications and Precautions: Metaraminol is contraindicated in patients with hypovolemia, within 14 days of MAO inhibitor therapy; peripheral or mesenteric thrombosis; pulmonary edema, cardiac arrest; untreated hypoxia, hypercapnea, and acidosis. Safe use during pregnancy (category D) not established. Use with caution in digitalized patients and those with hypertension, thyroid disease, diabetes mellitus, cirrhosis of liver, and history of malaria (may produce relapse).

Adverse/Side Effects: CNS: Apprehension, restlessness, headache, tremor, weakness, convulsions • CV: Precordial pain, palpitation, tachycardia, bradycardia, severe hypertension, dysrhythmias, cardiac arrest • Respiratory: Acute pulmonary edema • GI: Nausea, vomiting • Skin: Flushing, pallor, sweating, tissue necrosis, sloughing • Metabolic: Metabolic acidosis (hypovolemic patients), hyperglycemia.

Interactions: Metaraminol can be deactivated by alkaline solutions such as sodium bicarbonate. Concomitant use with ergot alkaloids, MAO inhibitors, or tricyclic

Metaraminol

antidepressants may cause an excessive vasopressor response. Phentolamine may decrease the vasopressor response.

Prehospital Considerations

- IV preparation: For adults, 15–100 mg may be dissolved in 500 mL of D_5W, NS, or other compatible IV fluid and titrated to maintain BP at a desired level.
- IV administration: IV flow rate will be prescribed by physician (usually, systolic BP is maintained at 80–100 mm Hg for previously normotensive patients; for previously hypertensive patients it is maintained at 30–40 mm Hg below the usual pressure).
- When infusion is to be discontinued, flow rate should be reduced gradually, and abrupt withdrawal avoided. Equipment for resuscitative therapy should be immediately available.
- Patients receiving drug IV must be constantly attended, with infusion flow rate being closely monitored. Changes in flow rate must be made cautiously, since the drug has cumulative effect and prolonged action.
- Care should be taken to avoid extravasation during IV infusion. Injury to local tissue and necrosis may result.
- Avoid exposure of drug to excessive heat, and protect it from light.
- During IV infusion, check BP every 5 min until it is stabilized at prescribed level, then every 15 min thereafter throughout therapy. Also note pulse rate and quality.
- Continue monitoring at regular intervals for several hours after infusion is complete.
- Metaraminol primarily works by stimulating the release of stored catecholamines. Patients who have been stressed by cardiac arrest or acute myocardial infarction have depleted stores of catecholamines, and the effects of metaraminol may be much less than expected.

Metaraminol

METHYLPREDNISOLONE

Class: Steroid

Trade Names: A-MethaPred, Solu-Medrol

Therapeutic Action/Pharmacodynamics:
Methylprednisolone is an intermediate-acting synthetic adrenal corticosteroid with similar glucocorticoid activity but considerably fewer sodium and water retention effects than hydrocortisone. Like the other steroids, its pharmacologic actions are vast and complex and, in medicine, have a wide range of uses.

Emergency Uses: To reduce the inflammation caused by severe anaphylaxis and asthma/COPD; to treat urticaria. *Adult dose:* 125–250 mg IV/IM. *Pediatric dose:* 1–2 mg/kg/dose IV/IM.

For treatment of suspected spinal cord injury: 30 mg/kg loading dose IV; followed by IV infusion of 5.4 mg/kg/hr for 23 hr.

Pharmacokinetics
Absorption: Peak effects in 4–8 days; duration is 1–5 weeks; half–life is 3.5 hr.
Metabolism: Metabolized in liver.
Elimination: HPA suppression in 18–36 hr.

Contraindications and Precautions: There are no major contraindications to using methylprednisolone in the management of acute anaphylaxis.

Adverse/Side Effects: CNS: Euphoria, headache, insomnia, confusion, psychosis, vertigo • CV: CHF, edema, hypertension • GI: Nausea, vomiting, peptic ulcer, abdominal distension • Musculoskeletal: Muscle weakness, delayed wound healing, muscle wasting, osteoporosis, aseptic necrosis of bone, spontaneous fractures
• Endocrine: Fluid retention, Cushingoid features, growth suppression in children, carbohydrate intolerance,

Methylprednisolone

hyperglycemia • Other: Cataracts, leukocytosis, hypokalemia, malaise, hiccups.

Interactions: Furosemide and thiazide diuretics may increase potassium loss. Phenytoin, phenobarbital, isoniazid, and rifampin may decrease the effectiveness of methylprednisolone and increase the metabolism of steroids.

Prehospital Considerations
- Give IM injection deep into large muscle (not deltoid).
- Provided in Mix-O-Vial from which solution is withdrawn and given by direct IV at a rate of 500 mg or fraction thereof over 60 sec or longer.
- IV administration to infants, children: Verify correct IV concentration and rate of infusion with physician.
- Methylprednisolone sodium succinate solution should be used within 48 hr after preparation.
- Most EMS agencies do not carry enough methylprednisolone for high-dose steroid therapy for spinal cord injuries. Systems that encounter, or are apt to encounter, spinal injuries should consider preparing a spinal injury pack with enough drug to handle a 220-pound (100-kg) adult.

METOCLOPRAMIDE

Class: Antiemetic
Trade Names: Clopra, Emex (Can), Maxeran (Can), Maxolon, Octamide, Pramin (Aus), Reclomide, Reglan
Therapeutic Action/Pharmacodynamics:
Metoclopramide is a potent central and peripheral dopamine receptor antagonist. It is structurally related to procainamide but has little antidysrhythmic or anesthetic activity. The exact mechanism of action is not clear, but it appears to sensitize GI smooth muscle to effects of

acetylcholine by direct action. It also increases the resting tone of the esophageal sphincter and the tone and amplitude of upper GI contractions. As a result, gastric emptying and intestinal transit are accelerated with little effect, if any, on gastric, biliary, or pancreatic secretions. Antiemetic action results from drug-induced elevation of CTZ threshold and enhanced gastric emptying.

Emergency Use: To relieve severe nausea and vomiting: *Adult dose:* 10–20 mg IM; 10 mg slow IV (over 1–2 min). *Pediatric dose:* 1–2 mg/kg/dose.

Pharmacokinetics
Absorption: Onset is 10–15 min IM, 1–3 min IV; peak effect in 1–2 hr; duration is 1–3 hr; half-life is 2.5–6 hr.
Distribution: Distributed to most body tissues, including CNS; crosses placenta; distributed into breast milk.
Metabolism: Minimally metabolized in liver.
Elimination: Excreted in urine, 5% in feces.

Contraindications and Precautions: Metoclopramide is contraindicated in patients with sensitivity or intolerance to metoclopramide, allergy to sulfite agents, history of seizure disorders, concurrent use of drugs that can cause extrapyramidal symptoms, pheochromocytoma, mechanical GI obstruction or perforation; history of breast cancer. Use with caution in patients with CHF, hypokalemia; renal dysfunction; GI hemorrhage; history of intermittent porphyria.

Adverse/Side Effects: CNS: Mild sedation (50% of patients), fatigue, restlessness, agitation, headache, insomnia, disorientation, extrapyramidal symptoms (acute dystonic type) • GI: Nausea, constipation, diarrhea, dry mouth • Other: Urticarial or maculopapular rash, glossal or periorbital edema, amenorrhea, impotence, altered drug absorption, hypertensive crisis (rare).

Interactions: Alcohol and other CNS depressants add to sedation. Anticholinergics and opiate analgesics may antagonize effect on GI motility. Phenothiazines may potentiate extrapyramidal symptoms. Hypertension may occur when metoclopramide is administered to patients taking MAO inhibitors.

Prehospital Considerations

- The injection form contains sodium metabisulfite as antioxidant. If patient has a history of allergy to sulfite agents, this product should be avoided.
- Store in light-resistant bottle at 15–30C (59–86F). Tablets are stable for 3 yr; solutions and injections, for 5 yr.
- Extrapyramidal symptoms are most likely to occur in children, young adults, and the elderly, and with high-dose treatment of vomiting associated with cancer chemotherapy. Report immediately the onset of restlessness, involuntary movements, facial grimacing, rigidity, or tremors. Have diphenhydramine available as an antidote.

METOPROLOL

Class: Beta blocker

Trade Names: Apo-Metoprolol (Can), Betaloc (Can), Lopressor, Minax (Aus), Novometoprol (Can), Nu-Metop (Can)

Therapeutic Action/Pharmacodynamics: Metoprolol is a beta-adrenergic blocking agent with preferential effect on beta$_1$ adrenoreceptors located primarily on cardiac muscle. At higher doses, metoprolol also inhibits beta$_2$ receptors located chiefly on bronchial and vascular musculature. It reduces heart rate and cardiac output at rest and during exercise; lowers both supine and standing BP, slows sinus rate, and decreases myocardial automaticity. Its antihypertensive action may be due to competitive antagonism of catecholamines at cardiac adrenergic neuron sites, drug-induced reduction of sympathetic outflow to the periphery, and to suppression of renin activity. Antianginal effect is like that of propranolol. Metoprolol and other beta blockers are cardioprotective in the period following an acute myocardial infarction.

Emergency Use: To reduce the incidence of ventricular fibrillation and other complications in patients who have recently suffered an MI (especially in those who did not receive fibrinolytic therapy). *Adult dose:* 5 mg slow IV every 5 min up to three times (if patient remains stable), resulting in a total dose of 15 mg. *Pediatric dose:* Not used.

Pharmacokinetics

Absorption: Onset is immediate; peak effect in 20 min; duration is 13–19 hr; half-life is 3–4 hr.
Distribution: Crosses blood-brain barrier and placenta; distributed into breast milk.
Metabolism: Extensively metabolized in liver.
Elimination: Excreted in urine.

Contraindications and Precautions: Metoprolol is contraindicated in patients in cardiogenic shock (BP less than 100 mm Hg), sinus bradycardia (less than 45 bpm), heart block greater than first degree (or PRI greater than 0.24), overt cardiac failure, and right ventricular failure secondary to pulmonary hypertension. It should not be used in patients with asthma or COPD in the prehospital setting. Use with caution in patients with impaired hepatic or renal function; cardiomegaly, CHF controlled by digitalis and diuretics; AV conduction defects; bronchial asthma and other bronchospastic diseases; history of allergy; thyrotoxicosis; diabetes mellitus; or peripheral vascular disease.

Adverse/Side Effects: CNS: Dizziness, fatigue, insomnia, increased dreaming, mental depression • CV: Bradycardia, palpitation, cold extremities, intermittent claudication, angina pectoris, CHF, intensification of AV block, AV dissociation, complete heart block, cardiac arrest • Respiratory: Bronchospasm (with high doses), shortness of breath • GI: Nausea, heartburn, gastric pain, diarrhea or constipation, flatulence • Skin: Dry skin, pruritus, skin eruptions • Other: Dry mouth and mucous membranes, hypoglycemia.

Interactions: Barbiturates and rifampin may decrease the effects of metoprolol. Cimetidine, methimazole, propylthiouracil, and oral contraceptives may increase effects of metoprolol. You may see additive bradycardic effects with digoxin. The effects of both metoprolol and hydralazine may be increased if used together. Beta agonists and metoprolol are mutually antagonistic. Verapamil may increase the risk of heart block and bradycardia.

Prehospital Considerations
- IV metoprolol may be given by direct IV undiluted at a rate of 5 mg over 60 seconds.
- Store at 15–30C (59–86F). Protect from heat, light, and moisture.
- Take apical pulse and BP before administering drug. Report to physician significant changes in rate, rhythm, or quality of pulse or variations in BP prior to administration.
- During IV administration, BP, heart rate, and ECG should be carefully monitored.
- Hypertensive patients with CHF controlled by digitalis and diuretics must be closely observed for impending heart failure: dyspnea on exertion, orthopnea, night cough, edema, distended neck veins.

Metoprolol

MIDAZOLAM

Class: Sedative

Trade Name: Hypnovel (Aus), Versed

Therapeutic Action/Pharmacodynamics: Midazolam is a short-acting parenteral benzodiazepine with CNS depressant, muscle relaxant, anticonvulsant, and anterograde amnestic effects. Its exact mechanism of action is unclear. Intensifies activity of gamma-aminobenzoic acid (GABA), a major inhibitory neurotransmitter of the brain, by interfering with its reuptake and promoting its accumulation at neuronal synapses. This calms the patient, relaxes skeletal muscles, and in high doses produces sleep. Like the other benzodiazepines, it has no effect on pain. Midazolam has considerably less muscle relaxant properties than diazepam.

Emergency Use: To induce sedation and amnesia prior to cardioversion and other painful procedures. *Adult dose:* 1.0–2.5 mg slow IV; 0.07–0.08 mg/kg IM (usual dose is 5 mg). *Pediatric dose:* 0.05–0.20 mg/kg IV; 0.10–0.15 mg/kg IM; 3 mg intranasal.

Pharmacokinetics

Absorption: Onset is 3–5 min IV, 15 min IM, 6–14 min intranasal; peak effects in 20–60 min; duration is less than 2 hr IV, 1–6 hr IM; half-life is 1–4 hr.

Distribution: Crosses blood-brain barrier and placenta.

Metabolism: Metabolized in liver.

Elimination: Excreted in urine.

Contraindications and Precautions: Midazolam is contraindicated in patients with intolerance to benzodiazepines, acute narrow-angle glaucoma, shock, coma, and acute alcohol intoxication. Use with caution in patients with COPD, chronic renal failure, CHF, and in the elderly.

Adverse/Side Effects: CNS: Retrograde amnesia, headache, euphoria, drowsiness, excessive sedation, confusion • CV: Hypotension • Eye: Blurred vision, diplopia, nystagmus, pinpoint pupils • GI: Nausea, vomiting • Respiratory: Coughing, laryngospasm (rare), respiratory arrest • Skin: Hives, swelling, burning, pain, induration at injection site, tachypnea • Other: Hiccups, chills, weakness.

Interactions: Alcohol, CNS depressants, and anticonvulsants potentiate CNS depression. Cimetidine increases midazolam plasma levels, increasing its toxicity. Midazolam may decrease the antiparkinsonism effects of levodopa. It also may increase phenytoin levels. Smoking decreases its sedative and antianxiety effects.

Prehospital Considerations

- Inject IM drug deep into a large muscle mass, not the deltoid.
- IV midazolam is given diluted to a concentration of 0.25 mg/mL in NS or D_5W. Avoid rapid injection, which may cause respiratory depression.
- IV administration to neonates, infants: Verify correct IV concentration and rate of infusion with physician.
- During IV infusion, inspect injection site for redness, pain, swelling, and other signs of extravasation.
- If the patient is premedicated with a narcotic agonist analgesic, the conscious sedation period may be marked by hypotension.
- Anterograde amnesia (dose related) correlates well with degree of drowsiness and is about the same as that for lorazepam. Most patients do not recall induction.
- In the obese patient, half-life is prolonged; therefore, duration of effects is prolonged (i.e., amnesia, postoperative recovery). Monitor vital signs for entire recovery period.
- Overdose symptoms include somnolence, confusion, sedation, diminished reflexes, coma, and untoward effects on vital signs.

Midazolam

- Prepare patient for the amnesia to prevent an upsetting postoperative period.
- Have resuscitative equipment and flumazenil (antidote) available prior to administering midazolam.

MILRINONE

Classes: Cardiac inotrope; vasodilator

Trade Name: Primacor

Therapeutic Action/Pharmacodynamics: Milrinone is a member of a new class of inotropic/vasodilator agents (same family as amrinone). It is a positive inotrope and vasodilator, with little chronotropic activity; mode of action and structure are different from digitalis and catecholamines as well as beta-adrenergic agents. Milrinone inhibits cyclic-AMP phosphodiesterase in cardiac and smooth vascular muscle. In therapeutic doses, milrinone increases cardiac contractility. Therefore, milrinone increases cardiac output and vascular resistance without increasing myocardial oxygen demand or significantly increasing heart rate.

Emergency Uses: Short-term management of CHF. *Adult dose:* Loading dose of 50 mcg/kg IV over 10 min followed by maintenance infusion of 0.375–0.75 mcg/kg/min IV. Milrinone is used occasionally to increase cardiac output and decrease systemic vascular resistance in pediatric septic shock. *Pediatric dose:* Loading dose of 50–75 mcg/kg IV followed by an IV infusion of 0.5–0.75 mcg/kg/min.

Pharmacokinetics

Absorption: Peak effect in 2 min; duration is 2 hr; half-life is 1.7–2.7 hr.

Elimination: 80–85% excreted unchanged in the urine.

Contraindications and Precautions: Milrinone is contraindicated in patients with a hypersensitivity to milrinone.

Use with caution in elderly patients, pregnancy (category C), and nursing mothers.

Adverse/Side Effects: CV: Increased ectopic activity, PVCs, ventricular tachycardia, ventricular fibrillation, supraventricular dysrhythmias, possible increase in angina symptoms, hypotension.

Interactions: Disopyramide may cause excessive hypotension.

Prehospital Considerations

- IV preparation and administration: Dissolve 20 mg of milrinone in 180 mL of NS or D_5W to yield 100 mcg/mL.
- Give loading dose of 50 mcg/kg IV over 10 min followed by maintenance dose.
- Dosages may be titrated for maximum hemodynamic effects.
- Do not administer to patients with known preexisting hypokalemia.
- Closely monitor cardiac status, ECG, pulse, blood pressure, and respirations during milrinone therapy.

MORPHINE

Class: Narcotic analgesic

Trade Names: Anamorph (Aus), Astramorph, Duramorph, Epimorph (Can), Infumorph, Kadian, Morphine, Roxanol, Statex

Therapeutic Action/Pharmacodynamics: Morphine is a natural opium alkaloid that acts on opiate receptors in the brain, providing both analgesia and sedation. Morphine is one of the most potent analgesics known, yet its hemodynamic properties make it extremely useful in managing patients with acute myocardial infarction and pulmonary edema. Its vasodilatory effects increase peripheral venous capacitance and reduce venous return. This reduces the cardiac workload and decreases myocardial oxygen demand, thus reducing infarction size in acute MI. In pulmonary edema, reducing preload significantly decreases pulmonary venous congestion.

Emergency Uses: To relieve moderate to severe pain. *Adult dose:* 2.5–15 mg IV; 5–20 mg IM/SC. *Pediatric dose:* 0.05–0.1 mg/kg IV; 0.1–0.2 mg/kg IM/SC.

To reduce venous return in acute MI and acute pulmonary edema. *Adult dose:* 1–2 mg every 6–10 min until desired response. *Pediatric dose:* Not used.

Pharmacokinetics

Absorption: Onset is immediate IV, 15–30 min IM/SC; peak effect in 20 min IV, 30–60 min IM/SC; duration is 2–7 hr.

Distribution: Crosses blood-brain barrier and placenta; distributed in breast milk.

Metabolism: Metabolized primarily in liver.

Elimination: 90% of drug and metabolites excreted in urine in 24 hr, 10% excreted in bile.

Contraindications and Precautions: Morphine is contraindicated in patients with hypersensitivity to opiates. Because it may mask symptoms, morphine should not be administered in the prehospital setting to patients with undiagnosed head injury or acute abdomen. Because of its vasodilatory effects, do not administer morphine to patients who are volume depleted or severely hypotensive. Do not use in patients with acute bronchial asthma, chronic pulmonary diseases, severe respiratory depression, and pulmonary edema induced by chemical irritants. Use with caution in very old, very young, or debilitated patients.

Adverse/Side Effects: Allergic: Pruritus, rash, urticaria, edema, hemorrhagic urticaria (rare), anaphylactoid reaction (rare) • CNS: Respiratory depression, euphoria, insomnia, disorientation, visual disturbances, dysphoria, paradoxic CNS stimulation (restlessness, tremor, delirium, insomnia), convulsions (infants and children); decreased cough reflex, drowsiness, dizziness, miosis. • CV: Bradycardia, palpitations, syncope; flushing of face, neck, and upper thorax; orthostatic hypotension • GI: Constipation, anorexia, dry mouth, biliary colic, nausea, vomiting, elevated transaminase levels • GU: Urinary retention or urgency, dysuria, oliguria, reduced libido or potency (prolonged use) • Other: Sweating, prolonged labor and respiratory depression of newborn, precipitation of porphyria • Overdosage: Severe respiratory depression (as low as 2–4/min) or arrest; pulmonary edema, deep sleep, coma; skeletal muscle flaccidity; cold, clammy skin; hypotension, bradycardia, cardiac arrest, marked miosis, hypothermia.

Interactions: CNS depressants, sedatives, barbiturates, alcohol, benzodiazepines, and tricyclic antidepressants may potentiate the CNS depressant effects. Use MAO inhibitors cautiously; they may precipitate hypertensive crisis. Phenothiazines may antagonize analgesia.

Prehospital Considerations

- Dosage for elderly or debilitated patients is lower than for adult.
- IV administration: Morphine may be given by direct IV, diluted in 5 mL of sterile water for injection, over 4–5 min.
- IV administration to neonates, infants, children: Verify correct IV concentration and rate of infusion/injection with physician.
- Before administering the drug, note respiratory rate, depth, and rhythm and size of pupils. Respirations of 12/min or below and miosis are signs of toxicity. Withhold drug and report to physician.
- Observe patient closely to be certain pain relief is achieved. Record relief of pain (using a pain scoring

system) and duration of analgesia for reference when dosage modification is being considered.

- Elevated pulse or respiratory rate, restlessness, anorexia, or drawn facial expression may indicate need for analgesia.
- Differentiate among restlessness as a sign of pain and the need for medication, restlessness associated with hypoxia, and restlessness caused by morphine-induced CNS stimulation (a paradoxic reaction that is particularly common in women and elderly patients).
- Monitor vital signs at regular intervals. Morphine-induced respiratory depression may occur even with small doses, and it increases progressively with higher doses (generally reaching maximum within 90 min following SC, 30 min after IM, and 7 min after IV administration).
- Nausea and orthostatic hypotension (with light-headedness and dizziness) most often occur in ambulatory patients or when a supine patient assumes the head-up position or in patients not experiencing severe pain.
- Closely observe the patient with increased intracranial pressure or with head injury. Morphine effects may obscure neurologic signs of further increase in intracranial pressure.
- Have naloxone available as an antidote prior to administration.
- Morphine is a Schedule II controlled substance.

NALBUPHINE

Class: Narcotic analgesic
Trade Name: Nubain
Therapeutic Action/Pharmacodynamics: Nalbuphine is a synthetic narcotic analgesic with both agonist and antagonist properties. Its analgesic potency is equal to that produced by

equivalent doses of morphine. On a weight basis, it produces respiratory depression about equal to that of morphine; however, in contrast to morphine, higher doses (greater than 10 mg) produce no further respiratory depression. Its antagonistic potency is approximately one-fourth that of naloxone.

Emergency Use: To relieve moderate to severe pain. *Adult dose:* 5 mg IV/IM/SC; repeat 2 mg doses as needed up to 20 mg. *Pediatric dose:* 0.10–0.15 mg/kg IV/IM/SC (rarely used).

Pharmacokinetics
Absorption: Onset is 2–3 min IV, 15 min IM; peak effect in 30 min IV; duration is 3–6 hr; half-life is 5 hr.
Distribution: Crosses placenta.
Metabolism: Metabolized in liver.
Elimination: Eliminated in urine.

Contraindications and Precautions: Nalbuphine is contraindicated in patients with a history of hypersensitivity to the drug. Like morphine, it should not be administered to patients with undiagnosed head injury or acute abdomen in the prehospital setting. Use with caution in patients with impaired respirations. Because it may reverse the effects of narcotics, use with caution in patients with narcotic dependency.

Adverse/Side Effects: CNS: Nervousness, depression, restlessness, crying, euphoria, dysphoria, distortion of body image, unusual dreams, confusion, hallucinations; numbness and tingling sensations, headache, miosis• CV: Hypertension, hypotension, bradycardia, tachycardia, flushing• Respiratory: Dyspnea, asthma, respiratory depression• GI: Abdominal cramps, bitter taste, nausea, vomiting• Hypersensitivity: Pruritus, urticaria, burning sensation• Other: Speech difficulty, urinary urgency, blurred vision.

Interactions: Alcohol and other CNS depressants add to CNS depression. Nalbuphine can cause withdrawal symptoms in narcotic-addicted patients.

Nalbuphine

Prehospital Considerations

- Nalbuphine may be given by direct IV undiluted at a rate of 10 mg over 3–5 min.
- IV administration to infants, children: Verify correct rate of IV injection with physician.
- Protect nalbuphine from light and store at 15–30C (59–86F) unless otherwise directed.
- Assess respiratory rate before drug administration. Withhold drug and notify physician if respiratory rate falls below 12.
- Nalbuphine may produce allergic response in persons with sulfite sensitivity.
- Administer with caution to patients with hepatic or renal impairment.
- Nalbuphine may produce drowsiness. Monitor ambulatory patients.
- Use of drug during labor and delivery may cause respiratory depression of newborn.
- Because of its antagonistic properties, nalbuphine makes it difficult for anesthesia personnel to provide a balanced narcotic anesthesia to patients who received the drug in the field. Thus, there is an increased emphasis on utilizing the traditional analgesics (morphine, meperidine) in prehospital care.

NALOXONE

Class: Narcotic antagonist

Trade Name: Narcan

Therapeutic Action/Pharmacodynamics: Naloxone, an analog of oxymorphone, is a pure narcotic antagonist, essentially free of agonistic (morphine-like) properties. Thus it produces no significant analgesia, respiratory depression, psychotomimetic effects, or miosis when administered in the absence of narcotics and possesses more potent narcotic antagonist action. Naloxone competes for and displaces narcotic molecules from opiate receptors in the brain. It is used mainly to reverse the respiratory depression associated with overdose of the following narcotic agents: morphine, heroin, methadone, codeine, paregoric, meperidine (Demerol), hydromorphone (Dilaudid), fentanyl (Sublimaze), hydrocodone (Percodan), nalbuphine (Nubain), propoxyphene (Darvon), pentazocine (Talwin), butorphanol (Stadol).

Emergency Uses: To reverse the effects of narcotic analgesics; to manage coma of unknown origin. *Adult dose:* 0.4–2.0 mg IV/IM, 2.0–2.5 times dose ET; may be repeated every 2–3 min up to 10 mg until respirations are restored. *Pediatric dose:* 0.01 mg/kg IV/IM, 2.0–2.5 times dose ET; may be repeated every 2–3 min up to 10 mg until respirations are restored.

Pharmacokinetics

Absorption: Onset and peak effects in less than 2 min IV, 2–10 min IM/ET; duration is 20–120 min; half-life is 60–90 min.
Distribution: Crosses placenta.
Metabolism: Metabolized in liver.
Elimination: Excreted in urine.

Contraindications and Precautions: Naloxone is contraindicated in patients with a hypersensitivity to the drug and in patients whose respiratory depression is due to nonopioid drugs. Safe use during pregnancy (other than labor) (category B) and in nursing mothers not established. Because naloxone may cause abrupt and complete reversal of the narcotic effects and the resulting withdrawal, use with caution in patients who are known or suspected narcotic addicts. This includes newborn infants of mothers with known or suspected narcotic dependence.

Naloxone

Adverse/Side Effects: Excessive dosage in narcotic depression: Reversal of analgesia, increased BP, tremors, hyperventilation, slight drowsiness, elevated partial thromboplastin time • Too rapid reversal: Nausea, vomiting, sweating, tachycardia.

Interactions: Naloxone may cause withdrawal symptoms in narcotic addicts. Use only enough to reverse respiratory depression.

Prehospital Considerations

- Naloxone may be given slowly by direct IV in 0.1–0.2 mg increments at 2–3-min intervals until desired narcotic reversal is achieved.
- Protect drug from excessive light. Store at 15–30C (59–86F).
- Duration of action of some narcotics may exceed that of naloxone; therefore, patient must be closely observed. Keep physician informed; repeat naloxone dose may be necessary.
- Narcotic abstinence symptoms induced by naloxone generally start to diminish 20–40 min after administration and usually disappear within 90 min.
- Monitor respirations and other vital signs.
- The goal of prehospital naloxone therapy is to reverse any respiratory depression. Large, onetime boluses can induce an opiate withdrawal reaction that can be difficult to manage (massive diarrhea, vomiting, runny nose, coughing, abdominal pain, and agitation).

NESIRITIDE

Classes: Cardiovascular agent; peptide hormone
Trade Name: Natrecor
Therapeutic Action/Pharmacodynamics: Nesiritide is a human B-type natriuretic peptide (hBNP), produced by

recombinant DNA, which mimics the actions of human atrial natriuretic hormone (ANH). ANH is secreted by the right atrium when atrial blood pressure increases. Nesiritide, like ANH, inhibits antidiuretic hormone (ADH) by increasing urine sodium loss by the kidney and triggering the formation of a large volume of dilute urine. Nesiritide binds to a cyclic nucleic acid, which results in smooth muscle cell relaxation. The drug also causes dilation of veins and arteries. It is effective in managing dyspnea at rest in patients with acute congestive heart failure (CHF).

Emergency Use: Acute treatment of decompensated CHF in patients who have dyspnea at rest or with minimal activity. *Adult dose:* 2 mcg/kg IV bolus followed by maintenance infusion of 0.01 mcg/kg/min. *Pediatric dose:* Not indicated.

Pharmacokinetics
Absorption: Onset in 15 min; duration is 1 hr; half-life is 18 min.
Elimination: Filtrated by kidneys.

Contraindications and Precautions: Hypersensitivity to nesiritide, patients with a systolic blood pressure less than 90 mm Hg, cardiogenic shock, patients with low cardiac filling pressures, patients who should not receive vasodilators, such as those with significant valvular stenosis, restrictive or obstructive cardiomyopathy, constrictive pericarditis, pericardial tamponade; pregnancy (category C). Use with caution in patients who are lactating, concurrent administration of ACE inhibitors or vasodilators. Safety and efficacy in pediatric patients have not been established.

Adverse/Side Effects: General: Headache, back pain, catheter pain, fever, injection site pain, leg cramps• CNS: Insomnia, dizziness, anxiety, confusion, paresthesia, somnolence, tremor• CV: Hypotension, ventricular tachycardia, ventricular extrasystoles, angina, bradycardia, tachycardia, atrial fibrillation, AV node conduction abnormalities • GI: Abdominal pain, nausea, vomiting • Respiratory: Cough, hemoptysis, apnea • Skin: Sweating, pruritus, rash • Special senses: Amblyopia.

Interactions: None.

Prehospital Considerations

- Monitor hemodynamic parameters (e.g., BP, HR, ECG) throughout therapy. Notify physician immediately if systolic BP is less than 90 mm Hg.
- Establish hypotension parameters prior to initiating therapy.
- Reduce the dose or withhold the drug if hypotension occurs during administration. Reinitiate therapy infusion only after hypotension is corrected. Subsequent doses following a hypotensive episode are usually reduced by 30% and given without a prior bolus dose.

NIFEDIPINE

Class: Calcium channel blocker

Trade Names: Adalat, Novo-Nifedin (Can), Procardia

Therapeutic Action/Pharmacodynamics: Nifedipine is a calcium channel blocking agent that selectively blocks calcium ion influx across cell membranes of cardiac muscle and vascular smooth muscle without changing serum calcium concentrations. It reduces myocardial oxygen utilization and supply and relaxes and prevents coronary artery spasm but has little or no effect on SA and AV nodal conduction with therapeutic dosing. Nifedipine decreases peripheral vascular resistance and increases cardiac output. Vasodilation of both coronary and peripheral vessels is greater than that produced by verapamil or diltiazem and frequently results in reflex tachycardia. Decreased peripheral vascular resistance also leads to a rise in peripheral blood flow, the basis for use of this drug in treatment of Raynaud's phenomenon. It has minimal effect on myocardial contractility. Nifedipine is a class IV antidysrhythmic.

Emergency Uses: To increase coronary artery perfusion in angina pectoris; to manage severe hypertension. *Adult dose:* 10–20 mg capsule SL/PO. *Pediatric dose:* Not used.

Pharmacokinetics
Absorption: Onset is 1–5 min SL, 5–20 min PO; peak effects in 20–30 min SL, 1–2 hr PO; duration is 2–5 hr; half-life is 2–5 hr.
Distribution: Distributed into breast milk.
Metabolism: Metabolized in liver.
Elimination: 75–80% excreted in urine, 15% in feces.

Contraindications and Precautions: Nifedipine is contraindicated in patients with known hypersensitivity to nifedipine and in hypotensive patients.

Adverse/Side Effects: CNS: Dizziness, light-headedness, nervousness, mood changes, weakness, jitteriness, sleep disturbances, blurred vision, retinal ischemia, difficulty in balance, headache• CV: Hypotension, facial flushing, heat sensation, palpitations, peripheral edema, MI (rare) • GI: Nausea, heartburn, diarrhea, constipation, cramps, flatulence• Musculoskeletal: Inflammation, joint stiffness, muscle cramps• Other: Sore throat, weakness, dermatitis, pruritus, urticaria, gingival hyperplasia, fever, sweating, chills, febrile reaction, nasal congestion, sexual difficulties, dyspnea, cough, wheezing• Overdosage: Prolonged systemic hypotension.

Interactions: Beta blockers may increase the likelihood of CHF, bradycardia, and asystole. Nifedipine may increase the risk of phenytoin toxicity.

Prehospital Considerations
- To administer nifedipine sublingually, make several puncture holes in the capsule before placing it under the tongue where it can be absorbed.
- Nifedipine should not be given within the first 1–2 wk following an MI.
- Management of a hypertensive emergency is a controversial issue. As a rule, high blood pressure is a chronic illness. If the blood pressure must be lowered because of end-organ changes, then labetalol or sodium nitroprusside should be used.
- Protect capsules from light and moisture; store at 15–25C (59–77F).
- Careful monitoring of BP during titration period is indicated. Severe hypotension may be produced, especially if patient is also taking other drugs known to lower BP. Withhold drug and notify physician if systolic BP is less than 90 mm Hg.
- Monitor the blood sugar in diabetic patients. Nifedipine has diabetogenic properties.

NIMODIPINE

Class: Calcium channel blocker

Trade Name: Nimotop

Therapeutic Action/Pharmacodynamics: Nimodipine is a calcium channel blocking agent that is relatively selective for cerebral arteries compared with arteries elsewhere in the body. This may be attributed to the drug's high lipid solubility and specific binding to cerebral tissue. It reduces vascular spasms in cerebral arteries during a stroke.

Emergency Use: To improve neurologic deficits due to spasm following subarachnoid hemorrhage from ruptured congenital intracranial aneurysms in patients who are in good neurologic condition. *Adult dose:* IV: For first 2 hr, administer 1.0 mg (approximately 15 mcg/kg) each hour; after 2 hr, increase to 2.0 mg (approximately 30 mcg/kg) each hour IV. *Pediatric dose:* Safety in children not established.

Pharmacokinetics
Absorption: Readily absorbed from GI tract; peak effect in 1 hr; half-life is 8–9 hr.
Distribution: Crosses blood-brain barrier; possibly crosses placenta; distributed into breast milk.
Metabolism: 85% metabolized in liver; 15% in kidneys.
Elimination: More than 50% excreted in urine; 32% in feces.

Contraindications and Precautions: None.

Adverse/Side Effects: CNS: Headache • CV: Hypotension • GI: Hemorrhage, mild, transient increase in liver function tests.

Interactions: Hypotensive effects may be increased when nimodipine is combined with other calcium channel blockers.

Prehospital Considerations
- Make a hole in both ends of the capsule with an 18-gauge needle and extract the contents into a syringe if patient is unable to swallow. Empty the contents into an enteral (if in use) tube and wash down with 30 mL of NS.
- Use only approved bags or glass bottles because nimodipine reacts with polyvinylchloride (PVC).
- Take apical pulse prior to administering drug and withhold it if pulse is below 60. Notify the physician.
- Monitor frequently for adverse drug effects, including hypotension, peripheral edema, tachycardia, or skin rash.
- Monitor frequently for dizziness or light-headedness in older adult patients; risk of hypotension is increased.

NITROGLYCERIN

Class: Nitrate

Trade Names: Anginine (Aus), Deponit, GTN-Pohl (Aus), Minitran, Nitradisc (Aus), Nitro-Bid, Nitrocap, Nitrocine, Nitrodisc, Nitro-Dur, Nitrogard, Nitroglyn, Nitroject, Nitrol, Nitrolate (Aus), Nitrolingual, Nitrong, Nitrostat, Transderm-Nitro (Aus), Tridil

Therapeutic Action/Pharmacodynamics: Nitroglycerin is an organic nitrate and potent vasodilator with antianginal, anti-ischemic, and antihypertensive effects. It relaxes vascular smooth muscle by unknown mechanism, resulting in dose-related dilation of both venous and arterial blood vessels. It also promotes peripheral pooling of blood, reduction of peripheral resistance, and decreased venous return to the heart. Both left ventricular preload and afterload are reduced, and myocardial oxygen consumption or demand is decreased. Therapeutic doses may reduce systolic, diastolic, and mean BP; heart rate is usually slightly increased.

Emergency Uses: To increase coronary artery perfusion and relieve chest pain in angina and acute myocardial infarction; to reduce preload in acute pulmonary edema. *Adult dose:* 0.4 mg SL, may repeat every 3–5 min up to 3 tablets; or 0.5–1 in (1.25–2.50 cm) ointment applied topically; or 0.4 mg (1 spray) SL spray up to 3 sprays/25 min. *Pediatric dose:* Not used.

Pharmacokinetics

Absorption: Onset is 1–3 min SL, 30 min transdermal; peak effect in 5–10 min SL; duration is 20–30 min SL, 3–6 hr transdermal; half-life is 1–4 min.

Distribution: Widely distributed; not known if distributes to breast milk.

Metabolism: Extensively metabolized in liver.

Elimination: Inactive metabolites excreted in urine.

Nitroglycerin

Contraindications and Precautions: Nitroglycerin is contraindicated in patients with hypersensitivity, idiosyncrasy, or tolerance to nitrates; patients taking sildenafil; severe anemia; head trauma, increased ICP; glaucoma (sustained release forms). Do not administer to patients in shock.

Adverse/Side Effects: CNS: Headache, apprehension, blurred vision, weakness, vertigo, dizziness, faintness • CV: Postural hypotension, palpitations, tachycardia (sometimes with paradoxical bradycardia), increase in angina, syncope, and circulatory collapse • GI: Nausea, vomiting, involuntary passing of urine and feces, abdominal pain, dry mouth • Skin: Cutaneous vasodilation with flushing, rash, exfoliative dermatitis, contact dermatitis with transdermal patch; topical allergic reactions with ointment: pruritic eczematous eruptions, anaphylactoid reaction characterized by oral mucosal and conjunctival edema • Other: Muscle twitching, pallor, perspiration, cold sweat; local sensation in oral cavity at point of dissolution of sublingual forms.

Interactions: Alcohol and antihypertensive agents may compound the hypotensive effects. Nitroglycerin may cause orthostatic hypotension when used in conjunction with beta blockers. Patients taking sildenafil are at risk for severe cardiac event.

Prehospital Considerations

General

- Approximately 50% of all patients experience mild to severe headaches following nitroglycerin. Assess patient and consult as needed with physician about analgesics and dosage adjustment.
- Transient headache usually lasts about 5 min after sublingual administration and seldom longer than 20 min. Assess degree of severity.
- Postural hypotension may occur even with small doses of nitroglycerin. Patient may complain of dizziness or

weakness due to postural hypotension. Supervision of ambulation may be indicated, especially with the elderly or debilitated patient.

- Use with caution in patients who have taken sildenafil (Viagra) in the last 6 hr because hypotension can result.
- Overdose symptoms include hypotension, tachycardia; warm, flushed skin becoming cold and cyanotic; headache, palpitations, confusion, nausea, vomiting, moderate fever, and paralysis. Tissue hypoxia leads to coma, convulsions, cardiovascular collapse. Death can occur from asphyxia.

Sublingual Tablet

- Instruct patient to sit or lie down upon first indication of oncoming anginal pain and to place tablet under tongue or in buccal pouch (hypotensive effect of drug is intensified in the upright position).
- Instruct patient to allow tablet to dissolve naturally and not to swallow until drug is entirely dissolved. Advise patient with dry mouth to take a sip of water or place 1 mL saline under the tongue before taking the nitroglycerin tablet.
- If pain is not relieved after 1 tablet, additional tablets may be taken at 5-min intervals, but not more than 3 tablets should be taken in a 15-min period. Taking more tablets than necessary can further decrease coronary blood flow by producing systemic hypotension.
- Any local burning or tingling from the sublingual form has no clinical significance.
- Always make sure that nitroglycerin tablets are fresh. The drug readily degrades upon exposure to air and light.

Sublingual Spray

- Do not shake canister. Spray preferably on or under tongue. Do not inhale spray.
- Spray may be repeated every 5 min for a maximum of 3 metered doses.
- Wait at least 10 seconds before swallowing.

Transdermal

- Using dose-determining applicator (patch) supplied with package, squeeze prescribed dose onto the applicator. Place patch with ointment-side down onto desired site. Using applicator, spread ointment in a thin, uniform layer to premarked 5.5 cm by 9 cm ($2\frac{1}{4}$ in by $3\frac{1}{2}$ in) square nonhairy skin surface (areas commonly used: chest, abdomen, anterior thigh, forearm). Cover with transparent wrap and secure with tape. Avoid getting ointment on fingers.
- Keep ointment container tightly closed and store in cool place.
- Before initiation of treatment with transdermal preparations, take baseline BP and heart rate, with patient in sitting position.
- Assess for and report blurred vision or dry mouth.
- Assess for and report the following topical reactions to drug administration: contact dermatitis from the transdermal patch; pruritus and erythema from the ointment.

NITROUS OXIDE

Class: General anesthetic

Trade Names: Dolonox (UK), Entonox (UK, Can, Aus), Nitronox

Therapeutic Action/Pharmacodynamics: Nitrous oxide (N_2O) is a general inhalation anesthetic and is the principal adjunct to anesthesia. It is an almost odorless and nonexplosive gas with relatively low anesthetic potency and muscle relaxant properties. It has strong analgesic properties. Nitronox is a blended mixture of 50% nitrous oxide and 50% oxygen that has potent analgesic effects. It is a self-administered CNS depressant whose effects quickly dissipate within ~2–5 min after cessation of administration. It is used in many situations to manage pain and, at the same time, reduce hypoxia.

Emergency Uses: To relieve pain of musculoskeletal origin (especially fractures), burns, suspected ischemic chest pain, and severe states of anxiety, including hyperventilation. *Adult dose:* Self-administered inhalation until pain is relieved or patient drops mask. *Pediatric dose:* Same as adult.

Pharmacokinetics
Absorption: Onset, peak effect, and duration are 2–5 min.
Distribution: Generally to all body areas.
Excretion: Rapidly eliminated via the lungs, with small amounts being eliminated through the skin and breast milk.

Contraindications and Precautions: Nitronox is contraindicated in a patient who cannot understand verbal instructions, who is intoxicated with alcohol or other drugs, or who has an altered mental status following a head injury. Do not use with patients with COPD for two reasons: (1) if they have hypoxic drive, the 50% oxygen may cause respiratory depression or arrest; (2) many COPD patients have blebs in their lungs, and nitrous oxide tends to diffuse into these closed spaces and cause swelling. Swollen blebs may rupture, causing a pneumothorax. For this same reason, do not administer Nitronox to patients with thoracic injuries, because a simple pneumothorax can be greatly worsened, or to patients with bowel obstruction.

Adverse/Side Effects: CNS: Dizziness, light-headedness, altered mental status, hallucinations • GI: Nausea and vomiting.

Interactions: Nitrous oxide can potentiate the effects of other CNS depressants such as narcotics, sedatives, hypnotics, and alcohol.

Prehospital Considerations
- Use nitrous oxide only in areas that are well ventilated.
- When used in the back of your ambulance, it is recommended that a scavenging system be in place.
- In countries where single-cylinder nitrous oxide/oxygen (Dolonox) systems are used, be sure that the equipment is kept above 40 degrees F as the nitrous oxide will assume the liquid state and oxygen only will be administered.

NOREPINEPHRINE

Class: Sympathomimetic
Trade Names: Levarterenol, Levophed, Noradrenaline
Therapeutic Action/Pharmacodynamics:
Norepinephrine is a direct-acting sympathomimetic amine identical to body catecholamine norepinephrine. It acts directly and predominantly on alpha-adrenergic receptors; little action on beta receptors except in heart (beta$_1$ receptors). Its main therapeutic effects are vasoconstriction and cardiac stimulation. It has powerful vasoconstrictor action on resistance and capacitance blood vessels. Peripheral vasoconstriction and moderate inotropic stimulation of heart result in increased systolic and diastolic blood pressure, myocardial oxygenation demand, coronary artery blood flow, and work of heart. Cardiac output varies reflexively with systemic BP.

Emergency Uses: To restore blood pressure in certain acute hypotensive states in patients refractory to other sympathomimetics; neurogenic shock. *Adult dose:* 0.5–30 mcg/min IV infusion titrated to BP. *Pediatric dose:* 0.01 mcg/kg/min (rarely used).

Pharmacokinetics
Absorption: Onset and peak effects are very rapid; duration is 1–2 min after termination of infusion.

Distribution: Localizes in sympathetic nerve endings; crosses placenta.
Metabolism: Metabolized in liver and other tissues by COMT and MAO.
Elimination: Excreted in urine.

Contraindications and Precautions: Norepinephrine is contraindicated as the sole therapy in hypovolemic states, except as a temporary emergency measure. Use with caution in patients with hypertension; hyperthyroidism; severe heart disease; in elderly patients; within 14 days of MAO inhibitor therapy; and in patients receiving tricyclic antidepressants.

Adverse/Side Effects: CNS: Headache, restlessness, anxiety, tremors, dizziness, weakness, insomnia • CV: Palpitation, hypertension, reflex bradycardia, fatal dysrhythmias (large doses) • Respiratory: Respiratory difficulty • Skin: Pallor, tissue necrosis at injection site (with extravasation) • With prolonged administration: Plasma volume depletion, edema, hemorrhage, intestinal, hepatic, and renal necrosis • Overdosage or individual sensitivity: Blurred vision, photophobia, hyperglycemia, retrosternal and pharyngeal pain, profuse sweating, vomiting, severe hypertension, violent headache, cerebral hemorrhage, convulsions.

Interactions: Alpha and beta blockers antagonize its pressor effects. Tricyclic antidepressants may potentiate its pressor effects.

Prehospital Considerations
• IV infusion of norepinephrine in a saline solution alone is not recommended. Dextrose (in distilled water or saline solution) is used to prevent oxidation and thus loss of potency. Usual dilution is a 4-mg ampule in 1,000 mL diluent to yield 4 mcg/mL.
• Do not use solution if discoloration or precipitate is present. Protect from light.

- Initial rate of infusion is 0.5–1.0 mcg/min; then titrated to maintain BP. An infusion pump is used. Consult medical director for specific titration guidelines.
- Risk of extravasation is reportedly reduced if infusion is administered through a plastic catheter inserted deep into vein.
- Flow rate must be constantly monitored. Check infusion site frequently (tape should not obscure injection site). Report immediately any evidence of extravasation: blanching along course of infused vein (may occur without obvious extravasation), cold, hard swelling around injection site.
- When therapy is to be discontinued, infusion rate is slowed gradually. Abrupt withdrawal should be avoided.
- Patient should be monitored constantly while receiving norepinephrine. Take baseline BP and pulse before start of therapy, then every 2 min from initiation of drug until stabilization occurs at desired level, then every 5 min during drug administration.
- In normotensive patients, it is recommended that flow rate be adjusted to maintain BP at low normal (usually 80–100 mm Hg systolic). In previously hypertensive patients, systolic is generally maintained no higher than 40 mm Hg below preexisting systolic level.
- In addition to vital signs, carefully observe and record mental status (index of cerebral circulation), skin temperature of extremities, and color (especially of earlobes, lips, nail beds).
- Be alert to patient's complaints of headache, vomiting, palpitations, dysrhythmias, chest pain, photophobia, and blurred vision as possible symptoms of overdosage. Reflex bradycardia may occur as a result of rise in BP.
- Continue to monitor vital signs and observe patient closely after cessation of therapy for clinical sign of circulatory inadequacy.

Norepinephrine

- Extravasation may require treatment with phentolamine (Regitine), an alpha adrenergic blocker. 5–10 mg should be diluted in 10 mL of NS and injected into the affected area.

OLANZAPINE

Classes: Antipsychotic; selective serotonin reuptake inhibitor

Trade Name: Zyprexa

Therapeutic Action/Pharmacodynamics: Antipsychotic activity is thought to be due to antagonism for both serotonin and dopamine receptors. Olanzapine may inhibit the CNS presynaptic neuronal reuptake of serotonin and dopamine. It also may antagonize alpha-adrenergic receptors, resulting in the adverse effect of orthostatic hypotension.

Emergency Uses: Management of psychotic disorders, treatment of bipolar disorder, acute agitation. *Adult dose:* 10 mg IM (reduce to 5 mg in elderly patients). *Pediatric dose:* Safety and effectiveness in children not established.

Pharmacokinetics

Absorption: Onset in 15 min IM; peak effect in 6 hr; half-life is 21–54 hr.

Distribution: 93% protein bound; secreted into breast milk of animals (human secretion unknown).

Metabolism: Metabolized in liver.

Elimination: Approximately 57% excreted in urine, 30% in feces.

Contraindications and Precautions: Do not use in patients with delirium due to dementia-induced psychosis. Hypersensitivity to olanzapine; abrupt discontinuation, coma, severe CNS depression; tardive dyskinesia; infants, pregnancy (category C), lactation. Use with caution in patients with known cardiovascular disease, neurologic disease, stroke, cerebrovascular disease, Parkinson disease, dementia; history of seizures, conditions that predispose to hypotension (i.e., dehydration, hypovolemia); history of syncope; history of breast cancer; diabetes mellitus; prostatic hypertrophy; closed-angle glaucoma; paralytic ileus; urinary retention; hepatic or renal impairment, concurrent use of hepatotoxic drugs, jaundice; predisposition to aspiration pneumonia; may increase risk of stroke in elderly patients with dementia; history of or high risk for suicide. Safety and effectiveness in children under 18 yr are not established.

Adverse/Side Effects: General: Weight gain, fever, back and chest pain, peripheral and lower extremity edema, joint pain, twitching, premenstrual syndrome • CNS: Somnolence, dizziness, headache, agitation, insomnia, nervousness, hostility, anxiety, personality disorder, hypertonia, tremor amnesia, euphoria, stuttering, extrapyramidal symptoms (dystonic events, parkinsonism, akathisia), tardive dyskinesia • CV: Postural hypotension, hypotension, tachycardia • Special senses: Amblyopia, blepharitis • GI: Abdominal pain, constipation, dry mouth, increased appetite, increased salivation, nausea, vomiting, elevated liver function tests • Metabolic: Hyperglycemia, diabetes mellitus • Urogenital: Premenstrual syndrome, hematuria, urinary incontinence, metrorrhagia • Respiratory: Rhinitis, cough, pharyngitis, dyspnea • Skin: Rash.

Interactions: May enhance hypotensive effects of antihypertensives. May enhance effects of other CNS active drugs, alcohol. Carbamazepine, omeprazole, rifampin may increase metabolism and clearance of olanzapine. Fluvoxamine may inhibit metabolism and clearance of olanzapine. St. John's wort may cause serotonin syndrome (headache, dizziness, sweating, agitation).

Olanzapine

Prehospital Considerations

- Monitor BP and HR periodically. Monitor temperature, especially under conditions such as strenuous exercise, extreme heat, or treatment with other anticholinergic drugs.
- Monitor for seizures, especially in older adults and cognitively impaired persons.
- Carefully monitor blood glucose levels if diabetic.
- Elderly patients with dementia-related psychosis treated with atypical psychotics (such as Zyprexa) are at increased risk of death, and thus this class of drugs should not be used.

OXYGEN

Class: Gas

Trade Name: Oxygen

Therapeutic Action/Pharmacodynamics: Oxygen is a tasteless, odorless, colorless gas necessary for life. Oxygen enters the body through the respiratory system and is transported to the cells by hemoglobin, found in the red blood cells. Oxygen is required for the efficient breakdown of glucose into a usable energy form. The administration of enriched oxygen increases the oxygen concentration in the alveoli, which subsequently increases the oxygen saturation of available hemoglobin.

Emergency Use: To manage any situation in which hypoxia is suspected. *Adult dose:* 100% if patient is hypoxic. *Pediatric dose:* Same as adult.

Pharmacokinetics

Absorption: Onset is immediate; peak effect within 1 min; duration is less than 2 min.

Contraindications and Precautions: There are no contraindications to oxygen. Use with caution in patients with chronic obstructive pulmonary disease who may have hypoxic drive. If these patients suffer respiratory depression from the enriched oxygen, perform positive pressure ventilation as needed. Never withhold oxygen from a hypoxic patient, regardless of the history or diagnosis. In a prolonged transport of a neonate, high concentrations of oxygen may damage the infant's eyes (retrolental fibroplasia). This is rarely a prehospital concern, but is a consideration. Oxygen delivered at a rate of greater than 6 L/min should be humidified to prevent drying of the mucous membranes of the upper respiratory tract. Use a pulse oximeter to monitor the oxygen saturation of hemoglobin. This is an easy, reliable indicator of your patient's oxygen delivery status.

Adverse/Side Effects: Respiratory: Dried mucous membranes, irritation of upper respiratory tract.

Interactions: Oxygen may increase the toxicity of certain herbicides (i.e., paraquat, diaquat) in patients who may have ingested these poisons. These chemicals are sometimes sprayed onto illicit agricultural products such as marijuana.

Prehospital Considerations: Use the oxygen delivery system indicated by the situation and desired concentration:

Device	Flow Rate	Concentration
Nasal cannula	1–6 L/min	24–44%
Simple face mask	8–10 L/min	40–60%
Venturi mask	4–12 L/min	24–50%
Partial rebreather	6–10 L/min	35–60%
Nonrebreather	6–15 L/min	60–90%
BVM with reservoir	10–15 L/min	40–90%
Demand valve	10–15 L/min	100%

Oxygen

OXYTOCIN

Class: Hormone

Trade Names: Oxytocin, Pitocin, Syntocinon

Therapeutic Action/Pharmacodynamics: Oxytocin is a synthetic, water-soluble polypeptide identical pharmacologically to the oxytocin secreted by the posterior pituitary. By direct action on myofibrils, it produces phasic contractions characteristic of normal delivery. Oxytocin also promotes milk ejection (letdown) reflex in the nursing mother, thereby increasing flow (not volume) of milk, and facilitates flow of milk during periods of breast engorgement. Uterine sensitivity to oxytocin increases during the gestation period and peaks sharply before parturition. Oxytocin is used to induce labor in selected cases.

Emergency Use: To control postpartum hemorrhage. *Adult dose:* 3–10 U IM following delivery of the placenta; 10–20 U in 1,000 mL of D_5W or NS IV infusion titrated to the severity of the bleeding. *Pediatric dose:* Not used.

Pharmacokinetics

Absorption: Onset is immediately IV; 3–7 min IM; duration is up to 1 hr IV, 2–3 hr IM; half-life is 3–5 min.
Distribution: Distributed throughout extracellular fluid; small amount may cross placenta.
Metabolism: Rapidly destroyed in liver and kidneys.
Elimination: Small amounts excreted unchanged in urine.

Contraindications and Precautions: Oxytocin is contraindicated prehospital prior to delivery of the baby and in patients with hypersensitivity to oxytocin. When administered prior to delivery, oxytocin may cause fetal hypoxia, fetal asphyxia, fetal dysrhythmias, and possible fetal intracranial bleeding.

Adverse/Side Effects: CNS: Subarachnoid hemorrhage, anxiety • CV: Postpartum hemorrhage, cardiac dysrhythmias, pelvic hematoma, hypotension, ECG changes,

PVCs, precordial pain, edema, hypertensive episodes, cardiovascular spasm and collapse • Respiratory: Dyspnea • GI: Nausea, vomiting • Hypersensitivity: Hypersensitivity leading to uterine hypertonicity, tetanic contractions, uterine rupture, anaphylactic reactions • Metabolic: Antidiuretic hormone effects leading to severe water intoxication and hyponatremia • Skin: Cyanosis or redness of skin.

Interactions: Vasoconstrictors can cause severe hypertension.

Prehospital Considerations

- Ensure that the baby and placenta have been delivered and that there is not an additional fetus in the uterus.
- Oxytocin should never be administered by more than one route at a time.
- During delivery, IM oxytocin is most easily injected deep into deltoid muscle. Massage injection site to assist quick absorption.
- When diluting oxytocin for IV infusion, rotate bottle gently to distribute medicine throughout solution.
- IV preparation: For postpartum bleeding, add 10–40 U of oxytocin to 1 L of D_5W or NS to give 10–40 mU/mL.
- Administer properly diluted IV solution by continuous infusion only.
- Unless otherwise directed by manufacturer, store oxytocin solution in refrigerator but do not freeze.
- The fundus should be checked frequently during the first few postpartum hours and several times daily thereafter.
- Incidence of hypersensitivity or allergic reactions is higher when oxytocin is given by IM or IV injection rather than by IV infusion (diluted solution).

Oxytocin

PANCURONIUM BROMIDE

Class: Non-depolarizing neuromuscular blocker

Trade Name: Pavulon

Therapeutic Action/Pharmacodynamics: Pancuronium is a synthetic derivative of curare used to facilitate endotracheal intubation. Pancuronium competes with acetylcholine at its receptor sites on the postsynaptic membrane. This results in paralysis of muscle fibers served by the neuromuscular junction. It is reported to be five times as potent as curare but produces little or no histamine release or ganglionic blockade and thus does not cause bronchospasm or hypotension. It does not cause an initial depolarization wave as does succinylcholine.

Emergency Use: To facilitate endotracheal intubation. *Adult dose:* 0.04–0.1 mg/kg IV. *Pediatric dose:* Same as adult.

Pharmacokinetics

Absorption: Onset is 30–45 sec; peak effect in 3–5 min; duration is 30–60 min; half-life is 2 hr.

Distribution: Well distributed to tissues and extracellular fluids; crosses placenta in small amounts.

Metabolism: Small amount metabolized in liver.

Elimination: Excreted primarily in urine.

Contraindications and Precautions: Pancuronium is contraindicated in patients with hypersensitivity to the drug or bromides. Use with caution in debilitated patients and those with myasthenia gravis, pulmonary, hepatic, or renal disease, fluid or electrolyte imbalance.

Adverse/Side Effects: CNS: Skeletal muscle weakness, respiratory depression • CV: Increased pulse rate and BP, ventricular extrasystoles, burning sensation along course of vein • GI: Salivation.

Interaction: Lidocaine, procainamide, beta blockers, magnesium sulfate, quinidine, verapamil, and other neuromuscular blockers enhance the neuromuscular

Pancuronium Bromide

blocking action of pancuronium. Diuretics may increase or decrease neuromuscular blockade. Lithium prolongs duration of neuromuscular blockade. Narcotic analgesics possibly add to respiratory depression. Succinylcholine increases the onset and depth of neuromuscular blockade. Phenytoin may cause resistance to or reversal of neuro-muscular blockade.

Prehospital Considerations

- Pancuronium bromide may be given by direct IV undiluted over 30–90 sec.
- Refrigerate at 2–8C (36–46F). Do not freeze.
- Observe patient closely for residual muscle weakness and signs of respiratory distress during recovery period. Monitor BP and vital signs.
- Peripheral nerve stimulator may be used to assess the effects of pancuronium and to monitor restoration of neuromuscular function.
- Have resuscitative equipment available prior to administration.
- Remember that pancuronium, like other neuromus-cular blockers, has no effect on mental status. Sedatives/hypnotics should be administered prior to administering pancuronium in patients who are not unconscious.

PHENOBARBITAL

Class: Anticonvulsant

Trade Name: Luminal

Therapeutic Action/Pharmacodynamics: Phenobarbital is a long-acting barbiturate. The sedative and hypnotic effects of barbiturates appear to be due primarily to inter-ference with impulse transmission of cerebral cortex by inhibition of the reticular activating system. Phenobarbital has no analgesic properties, and small doses may increase reaction to painful stimuli. CNS depression may range from mild sedation to coma, depending on dosage, route of administration, degree of nervous system excitability, and drug tolerance. Phenobarbital limits spread of seizure activity by increasing threshold for motor cortex stimuli. Barbiturates are habit forming.

Emergency Uses: To control seizures, status epilepticus, and acute anxiety attacks. *Adult dose:* 100–300 mg slow IV/IM. *Pediatric dose:* 6–10 mg/kg slow IV/IM.

Pharmacokinetics
Absorption: Onset is 3–30 min IV; peak effect in less than 30 min IV; duration is 4–6 hr; half-life is 2–6 days.
Distribution: 20–45% protein bound; crosses placenta; enters breast milk.
Metabolism: Oxidized in liver to inactivated metabolites.
Elimination: Excreted in urine.

Contraindications and Precautions: Phenobarbital is contraindicated in patients with sensitivity to barbiturates. Use with caution in patients with impaired hepatic, renal, cardiac, or respiratory function; history of allergies; elderly or debilitated patients; patients with fever; hyperthyroidism; diabetes mellitus or severe anemia; during labor and delivery, lactation; patients with borderline hypoadrenal function.

Adverse/Side Effects: CNS: Somnolence, nightmares, insomnia, hangover, headache, anxiety, thinking abnormalities, dizziness, nystagmus, irritability, paradoxic excitement and exacerbation of hyperkinetic behavior (in children); confusion or depression or marked excitement (elderly or debilitated patients); ataxia, CNS depression, coma, and death • CV: Bradycardia, syncope, hypotension • Respiratory: Respiratory depression • GI: Nausea, vomiting, constipation, diarrhea, epigastric pain

• Hypersensitivity: Rash, angioneurotic edema, fever, serum sickness, urticaria; hypoventilation, apnea, laryngospasm, bronchospasm, circulatory collapse • Injection site (extravasation): Thrombosis, gangrene transient pain, tenderness, redness; IV: coughing, hiccuping, laryngospasm • Other: Liver damage, hypocalcemia.

Interactions: Alcohol and other CNS depressants compound CNS depression. Phenobarbital may decrease absorption and increase metabolism of oral anticoagulants. It increases the metabolism of corticosteroids, oral contraceptives, anticonvulsants, and digitoxin, possibly decreasing their effects. Antidepressants potentiate the adverse effects of phenobarbital.

Prehospital Considerations

- Administer IM deep into large muscle mass; volume should not exceed 5 mL at any one site.
- Commercially prepared solutions for injection (sodium phenobarbital) may be diluted with most IV infusion solutions. If not absolutely clear, discard.
- IV preparation: Slowly introduce sterile water for injection into ampule with sterile syringe. Use at least 10 mL of diluent. Rotate ampule to hasten dissolving drug (may take several minutes). If solution is not clear in 5 min or if a precipitate remains, discard.
- IV administration: No greater than 60 mg/min. Administer reconstituted IV solution no later than 30 min after preparation.
- Extravasation of IV phenobarbital may cause necrotic tissue changes that may necessitate skin grafting. Frequently check the injection site.
- Patients receiving large doses should be closely observed for at least 30 min to ensure that sedation is not excessive.
- Keep patient under constant observation when drug is administered IV, and record vital signs at least every hour or more often if indicated.

Phenobarbital

- Barbiturates do not have analgesic action, and they may be expected to produce restlessness when given to patients with pain.
- The elderly or debilitated patient and children sometimes have paradoxical response to barbiturate therapy, i.e., irritability, marked excitement (inappropriate tearfulness and aggression in children), depression, and confusion. Be alert to unexpected responses and report promptly. Protect the elderly patient from falling, irrational behavior, and effects of depression (anorexia, social withdrawal).
- Barbiturates increase the metabolism of many drugs, leading to decreased pharmacologic effects of those drugs. Whenever a barbiturate is added to an established regimen of another drug, close observation for changes in effectiveness of the first drug is essential, at least during early phase of barbiturate use.

PHENYTOIN

Class: Anticonvulsant

Trade Names: Dilantin, Phenytex

Therapeutic Action/Pharmacodynamics: Phenytoin is a hydantoin derivative chemically related to phenobarbital. Its precise mechanism of anticonvulsant action is not known, but it appears to reduce the voltage, frequency, and spread of electrical discharges within the motor cortex, resulting in seizure activity inhibition. It also has class IB antidysrhythmic properties similar to those of lidocaine and tocainamide (also class IB agents). In abnormal tissue phenytoin causes a slight increase in AV conduction velocity depressed by digitalis glycosides, prolongs effective refractory period, suppresses ventricular pacemaker automaticity, and may slow conduction or cause complete block in abnormal ventricular fibers.

Emergency Uses: To control seizures, status epilepticus. *Adult dose:* 10–15 mg/kg slow IV. *Pediatric dose:* 8–10 mg/kg slow IV.

To convert dysrhythmias induced by digitalis toxicity. *Adult dose:* 100 mg slow IV (over 5 min) to a maximum loading dose of 1,000 mg. *Pediatric dose:* 3–5 mg/kg slow IV.

Pharmacokinetics
Absorption: Onset in 3–5 min; peak effect in 1–2 hr; half-life is 22 hr.
Distribution: 95% protein bound; crosses placenta; small amount in breast milk.
Metabolism: Oxidized in liver to inactive metabolites.
Elimination: Metabolites excreted by kidneys.

Contraindications and Precautions: Phenytoin is contraindicated in patients with hypersensitivity to hydantoin products. It is also contraindicated in patients with seizures due to hypoglycemia, sinus bradycardia, complete or incomplete heart block, and Adams-Stokes syndrome. Use with caution in patients with impaired hepatic or renal function; alcoholism, hypotension, heart block, brachycardia, severe myocardial insufficiency, impending or frank heart failure; elderly, debilitated, gravely ill patients; diabetes mellitus, hyperglycemia; respiratory depression.

Adverse/Side Effects: CNS: Nystagmus, drowsiness, ataxia, dizziness, mental confusion, tremors, insomnia, headache, seizures • CV: Bradycardia, hypotension, cardio-vascular collapse, ventricular fibrillation, phlebitis • Eye: Photophobia, conjunctivitis, diplopia, blurred vision • GI: Nausea, vomiting, constipation, epigastric pain, dysphagia, loss of taste, weight loss, hepatitis, liver necrosis • Metabolic: Fever, hyperglycemia, glycosuria, weight gain, edema • Skin: Maculopapular, urticarial, or morbilliform rash; bullous, exfoliative, or purpuric dermatitis; keratosis;

neonatal hemorrhage • Other: Acute renal failure, acute pneumonitis, pulmonary fibrosis, lymphadenopathy.

Interactions: Alcohol decreases phenytoin effects; other anticonvulsants may increase or decrease phenytoin levels. Phenytoin may decrease absorption and increase metabolism of oral anticoagulants; phenytoin increases metabolism of corticosteroids, oral contraceptives, and nisoldipine, thus decreasing their effectiveness. Amiodarone increases phenytoin levels; antituberculosis agents decrease phenytoin levels.

Prehospital Considerations

- IV administration: Give by direct IV 50 mg or fraction thereof over 1 min (25 mg/min in elderly or when used as antidysrhythmic). Usually, phenytoin is not given as a continuous infusion.
- During IV phenytoin administration, observe injection site frequently to prevent infiltration. Local soft tissue irritation may be serious, leading to erosion of tissues. Elderly women, especially those with peripheral vascular disease, seem to be at high risk.
- To minimize local venous irritation, each IV injection is followed with an injection of sterile saline through the same in-place catheter or needle.
- To reduce side effects with IV administration, lower doses than the usual adult range are given to geriatric, severely ill, or debilitated patients and to those with liver damage; and the flow rate is reduced to 50 mg over a 2–3-min period.
- A slightly yellowed injectable solution may be used safely. Precipitation may be caused by refrigeration, but slow warming to room temperature restores clarity. Do not administer unclear solution.
- Store phenytoin at 15–30C (59–86F) in tightly closed container. Protect from light.

- Margin between toxic and therapeutic IV doses is relatively small. Continuously monitor vital signs and symptoms during IV infusion and for an hour afterward. Watch for respiratory depression. If patient is elderly or has cardiac disease, constant observation and a cardiac monitor are necessary.
- Observe patient closely for neurologic side effects. Have on hand oxygen, atropine, vasopressor, assisted ventilation, and seizure precaution equipment (mouth gag, nonmetal airway, suction apparatus).
- Phenytoin must not be diluted with, or administered through, dextrose-containing solutions (i.e., D_5W).

PHYSOSTIGMINE

Class: Parasympathomimetic

Trade Name: Antilirium

Therapeutic Action/Pharmacodynamics: Physostigmine inhibits cholinesterase from breaking down acetylcholine. This results in increased acetylcholine levels at the receptor sites and a prolonging of parasympathetic effects. It is used as an antidote for anticholinergic overdose from drugs such as atropine and scopolamine and from plants containing anticholinergic agents such as belladonna. Since toxic levels of tricyclic antidepressants also cause cholinesterase inhibition, physostigmine is sometimes given for tricyclic overdoses. Tricyclic overdoses can cause serious cardiac conduction disturbances, resulting in a variety of dysrhythmias. By inhibiting cholinesterase, physostigmine causes a decrease in cardiac automaticity and conductivity, mucus secretion, and pupillary constriction by directly affecting the autonomic ganglia.

Emergency Uses: To reverse CNS and cardiac effects of tricyclic antidepressant overdose, to reverse CNS toxic effects of atropine, scopolamine, and similar anticholinergic drugs. *Adult dose:* 0.5–3 mg IV (not faster than 1 mg/min); repeat as needed. *Pediatric dose:* 0.01–0.03 mg/kg IV; may repeat every 15–20 min to maximum total dose of 2 mg.

Pharmacokinetics
Absorption: Readily absorbed from mucous membranes, muscle, subcutaneous tissue; onset is 3–8 min; duration is 0.5–5.0 hr; half-life is 15–40 min.
Distribution: Crosses blood-brain barrier.
Metabolism: Metabolized in plasma by cholinesterases.
Elimination: Excretion not fully understood; small amounts excreted in urine.

Contraindications and Precautions: Physostigmine is contraindicated in asthma, diabetes mellitus, gangrene, cardiovascular disease, and narrow-angle glaucoma. If excessive parasympathetic actions are seen, such as increased salivation, emesis, or bradycardia, reduce the dosage or administer atropine to antagonize the effects.

Adverse/Side Effects: Acute toxicity: Cholinergic crisis • CNS: Restlessness, hallucinations, twitching, tremors, sweating, weakness, ataxia, convulsions, collapse, headache • Respiratory: Respiratory paralysis, pulmonary edema • CV: Bradycardia, hypotension • Eye: Constricted pupils, twitching of eyelids, lacrimation, dimness and blurring of vision • GI: Increased urination and defecation.

Interactions: Anticholinergic drugs such as atropine, antidepressants, antihistamines, and phenothiazines can antagonize the effects of physostigmine.

Prehospital Considerations
- Physostigmine is rarely required in the prehospital setting.
- Physostigmine is given by direct IV undiluted at a slow rate, no more than 1 mg/min. Rapid administration and overdosage can cause a cholinergic crisis.

- Monitor vital signs and state of consciousness in patients receiving drug for atropine poisoning. Since physostigmine is usually rapidly destroyed, patient can lapse into delirium and coma within 1 to 2 hr; repeat doses may be required.
- Monitor closely for side effects related to CNS and for signs of sensitivity to physostigmine. Have atropine sulfate readily available for clinical emergency.
- When used parenterally or orally, the following symptoms indicate need to discontinue drug: excessive salivation, emesis, frequent urination, or diarrhea. Excessive sweating or nausea may be eliminated by dose reduction.

PRALIDOXIME

Class: Cholinesterase reactivator

Trade Names: 2-PAM, Protopam Chloride

Therapeutic Action/Pharmacodynamics: Pralidoxime reactivates the cholinesterase inhibited by phosphate esters by displacing the enzyme from its receptor sites. The free enzyme then can resume its function of degrading accumulated acetylcholine, thereby restoring normal neuromuscular transmission. Since it is more active against effects of anticholinesterase at the skeletal neuromuscular junction than at autonomic effector sites or in CNS respiratory center, atropine must be given concomitantly to block effects of acetylcholine and accumulation in these sites. Pralidoxime also detoxifies some organophosphates by direct chemical reaction. It is saved for severe organophosphate poisonings to reverse the respiratory depression and skeletal muscle paralysis.

Emergency Use: As antidote in treatment of poisoning by organophosphate. *Adult dose:* 1–2 g in 250–500 mL NS

infused over 15–30 min; or 1–2 g IM/SC if IV not feasible.
Pediatric dose: 20–40 mg/kg IV/IM/SC.

Pharmacokinetics

Absorption: Peak effect in 5–15 min IV, 10–20 min IM; half-life is 0.8–2.7 hr.

Distribution: Distributed throughout extracellular fluids; crosses blood-brain barrier slowly if at all.

Metabolism: Probably metabolized in liver.

Elimination: Rapidly excreted in urine.

Contraindications and Precautions: Pralidoxime is contraindicated in poisonings by the carbamate insecticide Sevin, inorganic phosphates, or organophosphates having no anticholinesterase activity. Do not use in patients with asthma, peptic ulcer, severe cardiac disease, or in patients receiving aminophylline, theophylline, morphine, succinylcholine, reserpine, or phenothiazines. Rapid IV administration may result in tachycardia, laryngospasm, and muscle rigidity. If used with large atropine doses, the effects of atropine may be seen much earlier than expected. Excitement and manic behavior may occur in patients immediately following recovery from unconsciousness.

Adverse/Side Effects: CNS: Dizziness, headache, drowsiness, muscular weakness • Eye: Blurred vision, diplopia, impaired accommodation • CV: Tachycardia, hypertension • GI: Nausea • With rapid IV: Tachycardia, laryngospasm, muscle rigidity.

Interactions: Respiratory depressants can potentiate the effects of pralidoxime. These include narcotics, phenothiazines, antihistamines, and alcohol. Pralidoxime should not be used with theophylline preparations.

Prehospital Considerations

• The initial treatment of organophosphate poisoning is atropinization. Following adequate atropinization, and in severe overdoses, pralidoxime should be considered.

- Always protect yourself and other rescuers when caring for the victims of organophosphate poisoning.
- Infusion should be stopped or IV rate reduced if hypertension occurs.
- It is difficult to differentiate toxic effects of organophosphates or atropine from toxic effects of pralidoxime. Be alert for these signs and report them immediately: reduction in muscle strength, onset of muscle twitching, changes in respiratory pattern, altered level of consciousness, increases or changes in heart rate and rhythm.
- Excitement and manic behavior reportedly may occur following recovery of consciousness. Observe necessary safety precautions.
- Pralidoxime is relatively short-acting. In patients with myasthenia gravis, overdosage with pralidoxime may convert cholinergic crisis into myasthenic crisis.

PROCAINAMIDE

Class: Antidysrhythmic

Trade Names: Procan, Procanbid, Promine, Pronestyl

Therapeutic Action/Pharmacodynamics: Procainamide is an amide analog of procaine hydrochloride with cardiac actions similar to those of quinine. It is a Class Ia antidysrhythmic agent that depresses the excitability of the myocardium to electrical stimulation and reduces conduction velocity in the atria, ventricles, and His-Purkinje system. Procainamide increases the duration of the refractory period, especially in the atria. It also produces a slight change in contractility of cardiac muscle and cardiac output and suppresses automaticity of His-Purkinje ventricular muscle. It can produce peripheral vasodilaton and hypotension, especially with IV use.

Emergency Use: To convert ventricular fibrillation and pulseless ventricular tachycardia refractory to lidocaine to sinus rhythm. *Adult dose:* 20–30 mg/min IV infusion up to 17 mg/kg loading dose. Maintenance dose is 1–4 mg/min. *Pediatric dose:* 15 mg/kg IV/IO over 30–60 min.

Pharmacokinetics

Absorption: Onset is 10–30 min; peak effect in 15–60 min; duration is 3–6 hr; half-life is 3 hr.

Distribution: Distributed to CSF, liver, spleen, kidney, brain, and heart; crosses placenta; distributed into breast milk.

Metabolism: Metabolized in liver to N-acetylprocainamide (NAPA), an active metabolite (30–60% metabolized to NAPA).

Elimination: Excreted in urine.

Contraindications and Precautions: Procainamide is contraindicated in myasthenia gravis; hypersensitivity to procainamide or procaine; complete AV block, second- and third-degree AV block unassisted by pacemaker. Use with caution in patients with hypotension, cardiac enlargement, CHF, MI, coronary occlusion, ventricular dysrhythmia from digitalis intoxication, hepatic or renal insufficiency, electrolyte imbalance, bronchial asthma.

Adverse/Side Effects: CNS: Dizziness, psychosis • CV: Severe hypotension, pericarditis, ventricular fibrillation, AV block, tachycardia, flushing • GI: Nausea, vomiting, diarrhea, anorexia • Hematologic: Thrombocytopenia • Hypersensitivity: Fever, muscle and joint pain, angioneurotic edema, maculopapular rash, pruritus • Other: Pleuritic pain, pleural effusion, erythema, skin rash, myalgia, fever.

Interactions: Other antidysrhythmics add to therapeutic and toxic effects; anticholinergic agents compound anticholinergic effects; antihypertensives add to hypotensive effects; cimetidine may increase procainamide and NAPA levels with increase in toxicity.

Prehospital Considerations

- When procainamide is given direct IV, dilute each 100 mg with 10 mL of D_5W or sterile water for injection. When procainamide is given by IV infusion, add 1 g of procainamide to 250–500 mL of D_5W solution. Yields 4 mg/mL in 250 mL or 2 mg/mL in 500 mL.
- Procainamide administration by IV infusion pump requires constant monitoring to maintain desired flow rate. Keep patient in supine position. Be alert to signs of too rapid administration: irregular pulse, tight feeling in chest, flushed face, headache, loss of consciousness, shock, cardiac arrest.
- Procainamide solution is stable for 24 hr at room temperature and for 7 days under refrigeration at 2–8C (36–46F). Avoid freezing the solution. Refrigeration will retard color changes in solution. Slight yellowing does not alter drug potency, but discard solution if it is markedly discolored or precipitated.
- Patients at particular risk for adverse effects are those with severe heart, hepatic, or renal disease and hypotension.
- Monitor the patient's ECG and BP continuously during IV drug administration.
- IV drug is temporarily discontinued when dysrhythmia is interrupted; severe toxic effects are present; QRS complex is excessively widened (greater than 50%); PR interval is prolonged; or BP drops 15 mm Hg or more. Obtain rhythm strip and notify physician.

Procainamide

PROCHLORPERAZINE

Class: Antiemetic

Trade Names: Compazine, Prochlorparazine (Can), Prorazin (Can), Stemetil (Can)

Therapeutic Action/Pharmacodynamics: Prochlorperazine is a phenothiazine derivative with actions, contraindications, and interactions similar to those of chlorpromazine. It has greater extrapyramidal effects and antiemetic potency but fewer sedative, hypotensive, and anticholinergic effects than chlorpromazine. It does not prevent vertigo and motion sickness like many of the other phenothiazines. In addition, prochlorperazine has weak anticholinergic properties.

Emergency Uses: To relieve severe nausea and vomiting; to manage acute psychosis. *Adult dose:* 5–10 mg IV/IM. *Pediatric dose:* More than 10 kg or older than 2 yr: 0.13 mg/kg IV/IM/PR (rarely used).

Pharmacokinetics

Absorption: Onset is 10–20 min IV/IM, 60 min PR; duration is up to 12 hr IM, 3–4 hr PR.

Distribution: Crosses placenta; distributed into breast milk.

Metabolism: Metabolized in liver.

Elimination: Excreted in urine.

Contraindications and Precautions: Prochlorperazine is contraindicated in patients with hypersensitivity to phenothiazines and in patients who are comatose or severely depressed. Use with caution in patients with previously diagnosed breast cancer, and in children with acute illness or dehydration.

Adverse/Side Effects: CNS: Drowsiness, dizziness, extrapyramidal reactions (akathisia, dystonia, or parkinsonism), persistent tardive dyskinesia, acute catatonia, sedation • CV: Hypotension, tachycardia • Eyes: Photosensitivity, blurred vision • Skin: Cholestatic jaundice.

Interactions: Alcohol and other CNS depressants increase CNS depression. Phenobarbital increases the metabolism of prochlorperazine. Concomitant administration of phenylpropanolamine poses the possibility of sudden death. Tricyclic antidepressants intensify its hypotensive and anticholinergic effects and decrease the seizure threshold, so the anticonvulsant dosage may need to be increased.

Prehospital Considerations

- The incidence of extrapyramidal symptoms appears to be higher with prochlorperazine than with other phenothiazines. Have diphenhydramine available prior to administration.
- Dosage for elderly, emaciated patients and for children should be advanced slowly.
- Avoid skin contact with oral concentrate or injection solution because of possibility of contact dermatitis.
- IM injection in adults should be made deep into the upper outer quadrant of the buttock. Do not mix IM solution in the same syringe with other agents. Follow agency policy regarding IM injection site for children.
- IV administration: Give direct IV by diluting in D_5W, NS, or other compatible diluent to a concentration of 1 mg/mL and give at a maximum rate of 5 mg/min.
- Slight yellowing does not appear to alter potency; however, markedly discolored solutions should be discarded. Protect drug from light; do not freeze. Store at temperature between 15 and 30C (59 and 86F) unless otherwise instructed by manufacturer.
- Postoperative patients who have received prochlorperazine may have depressed cough reflex and should be carefully positioned to prevent aspiration of vomitus.

- Most elderly and emaciated patients and children, especially those with dehydration or acute illness, appear to be particularly susceptible to extrapyramidal effects. Be alert to onset of symptoms: in early therapy watch for pseudoparkinson's and acute dyskinesia.
- Keep in mind that the antiemetic effect may mask toxicity of other drugs or make it difficult to diagnose conditions with a primary symptom of nausea, such as intestinal obstruction and increased intracranial pressure.
- It has been reported that although the patient is not responsive during acute catatonia (side effect), everything that happens during the episode can be recalled. Approach patient accordingly.
- Be alert to signs: red, dry, hot skin; full bounding pulse; dilated pupils; dyspnea; confusion; temperature over 40.6C (105F); elevated BP. Inform physician and institute measures to reduce body temperature rapidly.
- Prochlorperazine is rarely used in children because of their tendency to develop extrapyramidal system symptoms with even low dosages.

PROMETHAZINE

Class: Antiemetic

Trade Names: Anergan, Histantil (Can), Pentazine, Phenameth, Phenergan, Phenoject-50, Promethegan, Prorex, Prothazine, V-Gan

Therapeutic Action/Pharmacodynamics:
Promethazine is a long-acting derivative of phenothiazine with marked antihistaminic activity and prominent sedative, amnesic, antiemetic, and anti–motion sickness actions. Unlike other

phenothiazine derivatives, it is relatively free of extrapyramidal side effects; however, in high doses it carries same potential for toxicity. In common with other antihistamines, exerts antiserotonin, anticholinergic, and local anesthetic action. Antiemetic action thought to be due to depression of CTZ in medulla.

Emergency Uses: To relieve nausea and vomiting, motion sickness; to potentiate the effects of analgesics; to induce sedation. *Adult dose:* 12.5–25.0 mg IV/IM/PR. *Pediatric dose:* 0.5 mg/kg IV/IM/PR.

Pharmacokinetics

Absorption: Onset is 20 min PR/IM, 5 min IV; duration is 2–8 hr.
Distribution: Crosses placenta.
Metabolism: Metabolized in liver.
Elimination: Slowly excreted in urine and feces.

Contraindications and Precautions: Promethazine is contraindicated in patients with hypersensitivity to phenothiazines, nursing mothers, newborn or premature infants, acutely ill or dehydrated children. Use with caution in patients with impaired hepatic function, cardiovascular disease, asthma, acute or chronic respiratory impairment (particularly in children), hypertension; elderly or debilitated patients.

Adverse/Side Effects: Acute toxicity: Deep sleep, coma, convulsions, cardiorespiratory symptoms, extrapyramidal reactions, nightmares (in children), CNS stimulation, abnormal movements, respiratory depression; toxic potential as for other phenothiazines • CNS: Sedation drowsiness, confusion, dizziness, disturbed coordination, restlessness, tremors • CV: Transient mild hypotension or hypertension • GI: Anorexia, nausea, vomiting, constipation • Other: Photosensitivity, irregular respiration, blurred vision, urinary retention; dry mouth, nose, or throat.

Interactions: Alcohol and other CNS depressants add to CNS depression and anticholinergic effects.

Prehospital Considerations

- Inspect parenteral drug before preparation. Discard if it is darkened or contains precipitate.
- IM injection is made deep into large muscle mass. Aspirate carefully before injecting drug. Intra-arterial injection can cause arterial or arteriolar spasm, with resultant gangrene. Subcutaneous injection (also contraindicated) can cause chemical irritation and necrosis. Rotate injection sites and observe daily.
- IV administration: IV promethazine in concentrations of 25 mg/mL or less may be given by direct IV undiluted over 2 min. More concentrated preparations should be diluted in NS to yield no more than 25 mg/mL.
- Store in tight, light-resistant container at 15–30C (59–86F) unless otherwise directed.
- Antiemetic action may mask symptoms of unrecognized disease and signs of drug overdosage as well as dizziness, vertigo, or tinnitus associated with toxic doses of aspirin or other ototoxic drugs.
- Patients in pain may develop involuntary movements of upper extremities following parenteral adminis-tration. These symptoms usually disappear after pain is controlled.
- Respiratory function should be monitored in patients with respiratory problems, particularly children. Promethazine may suppress cough reflex and cause thickening of bronchial secretions.
- Have diphenhydramine available in case extrapyramidal symptoms appear.

PROPAFANONE

Class: Antidysrhythmic

Trade Name: Rythmol

Therapeutic Action/Pharmacodynamics: Propafanone is a class IC antidysrhythmic drug with a direct stabilizing action on myocardial membranes. It reduces spontaneous automaticity. The rate of single and multiple PVCs is decreased by appropriate dose and concentration of propafanone. In addition, it suppresses ventricular tachycardia. Propafanone, like other class IC antidysrhythmics, exerts a negative inotropic effect on the myocardium. It also has nonselective beta-blocking properties.

Emergency Use: To convert ventricular and supraventricular dysrhythmias in patients without structural heart disease. *Adult dose:* 150–300 mg PO every 8 hr. IV dose is 1–2 mg/kg administered at 10 mg/min.

Pharmacokinetics

Absorption: Readily absorbed from GI tract; peak effect in 3.5 hr; half-life is 5–8 hr.

Distribution: 97% protein-bound, highest concentrations in the lung. Crosses placenta, distributed into breast milk.

Metabolism: Extensively metabolized in the liver.

Elimination: 18.5–38% of dose excreted in urine as metabolites.

Contraindications and Precautions: Propafanone is contraindicated in patients with uncontrolled CHF, cardiogenic shock, sinoatrial, AV, or intraventricular disorders (e.g., sick sinus node syndrome, AV block) without a pacemaker; bradycardia, marked hypotension, bronchospastic disorders; electrolyte imbalances; hypersensitivity to propafanone; non-life-threatening dysrhythmias, chronic bronchitis, emphysema, nursing mothers. Use with caution in patients with CHF, AV block, hepatic/renal impairment; in elderly patients; and during pregnancy. Safety and efficacy in children have not been established.

Adverse/Side Effects: CNS: Blurred vision, dizziness, paresthesias, fatigue, somnolence, vertigo, and headache • CV: Arrhythmias, ventricular tachycardia, hypotension, bundle branch block, AV block, complete heart block, sinus arrest, CHF, bradycardia • GI: Nausea, abdominal discomfort, constipation, vomiting, dry mouth, taste alterations, cholestatic hepatitis • Other: Rash.

Interactions: Amiodarone and quinidine increase the levels and toxicity of propafanone. May increase levels and toxicity of tricyclic antidepressants, cyclosporine, digoxin, beta blockers, theophylline, and warfarin. Phenobarbital decreases levels of propafanone.

Prehospital Considerations

- IV use of propafanone is not approved in the United States.
- Dosage is usually initiated with 150 mg every 8 hr and may be increased at 3–4 day intervals to a maximum of 300 mg every 8 hr.
- Dosage increments should be more gradual in elderly patients or in those with previous extensive myocardial damage.
- Dosage reduction should be considered with significant widening of the QRS complex or development of second- or third-degree AV block.
- With severe liver dysfunction, significant dose reduction is warranted.
- Monitor cardiovascular status frequently (e.g., ECG, Holter monitor) to determine effectiveness of drug and development of new or worsened arrhythmias.
- Development of second- or third-degree AV block after initiation of therapy requires dosage reduction or discontinuation of the drug.

- Advise patients to report any of the following: chest pain, palpitations, blurred or abnormal vision, dyspnea, or signs and symptoms of infection.
- Advise patients on concurrent warfarin therapy to report unusual bleeding or bruising.
- Instruct patients to monitor radial pulse daily and report decreased heart rate or development of an abnormal heartbeat.
- Alert elderly or debilitated patients to possibility of developing dizziness and need for caution with ambulation.

PROPOFOL

Class: Sedative-hypnotic

Trade Name: Diprivan

Therapeutic Action/Pharmacodynamics: Propofol is a short-acting sedative-hypnotic that produces anesthesia and deep sedation.

Emergency Use: As a short-acting anesthetic prior to initiating a painful procedure. *Adult dose:* 2–2.5 mg/kg (40 mg every 10 sec until onset). Maintenance 100–200 mcg/kg/min intermittent bolus: increments of 20–50 mg as needed. *Pediatric dose:* 2.5–3.5 mg/kg over 20–30 sec.

Pharmacokinetics

Absorption: Onset within 1 min; duration is 6–10 minutes; half-life is 5–12 hr.

Distribution: Highly lipophilic, crosses placenta, excreted in breast milk.

Metabolism: Extensively metabolized in the liver.

Elimination: Approximately 88% of the dose is recovered in the urine as metabolites.

Contraindications and Precautions: Hypersensitivity to propofol or propofol emulsion, which contain soybean oil and egg phosphatide; obstetrical procedures; patients with increased intracranial pressure or impaired cerebral circulation; pregnancy (category B), lactation. Do not use for conscious sedation in children less than 3 yr old. Use with caution in patients with severe cardiac or respiratory disorders or history of epilepsy or seizures.

Adverse/Side Effects: CNS: Headache, dizziness, twitching, bucking, jerking, thrashing, clonic/myoclonic movements • Special senses: Decreased intraocular pressure • CV: Hypotension, ventricular asystole (rare) • GI: Vomiting, abdominal cramping • Respiratory: Cough, hiccups, apnea • Other: Pain at injection site.

Interactions: Concurrent continuous infusions of propofol and alfentanil produce higher plasma levels of alfentanil than expected. CNS depressants cause additive CNS depression.

Prehospital Considerations
- Use strict aseptic technique to prepare propofol for injection; drug emulsion supports rapid growth of microorganisms.
- Inspect ampules and vials for particulate matter and discoloration. Discard if either is noted.
- Shake well before use. Inspect for separation of the emulsion. Do not use if there is evidence of separation of phases of the emulsion.
- Monitor hemodynamic status and assess for dose-related hypotension.
- Take seizure precautions. Tonic-clonic seizures have occurred following general anesthesia with propofol.
- Be alert to the potential for drug-induced excitation (e.g., twitching, tremor, hyperclonus) and take appropriate safety measures.
- Provide comfort measures; pain at the injection site is quite common especially when small veins are used.

Propofol

PROPRANOLOL

Class: Beta blocker

Trade Names: Apo-Propranolol (Can), Betachron, Deralin (Aus), Detensol (Can), Inderal, Novopranol (Can)

Therapeutic Action/Pharmacodynamics: Propranolol is a nonselective beta blocker of both cardiac and bronchial adrenoreceptors that competes with epinephrine and nor-epinephrine for available beta-receptor sites. It blocks cardiac effects of beta-adrenergic stimulation; as a result, it reduces heart rate, myocardial irritability (Class II anti-dysrhythmic) and force of contraction, depresses auto-maticity of sinus node and ectopic pacemaker, and decreases AV and intraventricular conduction velocity. In higher doses, it exerts direct quinidine-like effects that depress cardiac function. Propanolol lowers both supine and standing blood pressures in hypertensive patients. Its hypotensive effect is associated with decreased cardiac output and suppressed renin activity, as well as beta blockade. It also decreases platelet aggregation. The mechanism of antimigraine action is unknown but thought to be related to inhibition of cerebral vasodilation and arteriolar spasms.

Emergency Uses: To convert ventricular fibrillation and pulseless ventricular tachycardia refractory to lidocaine and bretylium; to convert selected supraventricular tachy-dysrhythmias. *Adult dose:* 1–3 mg slow IV (over 2–5 min), not to exceed 1 mg/min. May repeat dose in 2 min to total dose of 0.1 mg/kg. *Pediatric dose:* 0.01 mg/kg slow IV.

Pharmacokinetics

Absorption: Onset in less than 2 min; peak effect in 15 min; duration is 2–6 hr; half-life is 2.3 hr.

Distribution: Widely distributed including CNS, placenta, and breast milk.

Metabolism: Almost completely metabolized in liver.
Elimination: 90–95% excreted in urine as metabolites;
1–4% excreted in feces.

Contraindications and Precautions: Propranolol is contraindicated in patients with greater than first-degree heart block, CHF, right ventricular failure secondary to pulmonary hypertension, sinus bradycardia, cardiogenic shock, significant aortic or mitral valvular disease, bronchial asthma or bronchospasm, severe COPD, allergic rhinitis during pollen season. Avoid concurrent use with adrenergic-augmenting psychotropic drugs or within 2 wk of MAO inhibition therapy. Safe use during pregnancy (category C) and in nursing mothers is not established. Use with caution in patients with peripheral arterial insufficiency; history of systemic insect sting reaction; patients prone to nonallergenic bronchospasm (e.g., chronic bronchitis, emphysema); major surgery; renal or hepatic impairment; diabetes mellitus; patients prone to hypoglycemia; myasthenia gravis; Wolff-Parkinson-White syndrome.

Adverse/Side Effects: Allergic: Erythematous, psoriasis-like eruptions; pruritus; fever; pharyngitis; respiratory distress • CNS: Drug-induced psychosis, sleep disturbances, depression, confusion, agitation, giddiness, lightheadedness, fatigue, vertigo, syncope, weakness, drowsiness, insomnia, vivid dreams, visual hallucinations, delusions, reversible organic brain syndrome • CV: Palpitation, profound bradycardia, AV heart block, cardiac standstill, hypotension, angina pectoris, tachydysrhythmia, acute CHF, peripheral arterial insufficiency resembling Raynaud's disease, myotonia, paresthesia of hands • Eye/ear: Dry eyes (gritty sensation), visual disturbances, conjunctivitis, tinnitus, hearing loss, nasal stuffiness • GI: Dry mouth, cheilostomatitis, nausea, vomiting, heartburn, diarrhea, constipation, flatulence, abdominal cramps, mesenteric arterial thrombosis, ischemic colitis • Hematologic: Transient eosinophilia, hypoglycemia, hyperglycemia, hypocalcemia (patients with hyperthyroidism) • Respiratory: Dyspnea, laryngospasm, bronchospasm • Skin: Hyperkeratoses of scalp, palms, feet; nail changes; dry skin • Other: Pancreatitis, weight gain, impotence or decreased libido, cold extremities, leg fatigue, arthralgia.

Interactions: Phenothiazines have additive hypotensive effects. Beta-adrenergic agonists (e.g., albuterol) antagonize effects. Atropine and tricyclic antidepressants block bradycardia. Diuretics and other hypotensive agents increase hypotension. High doses of tubocurarine may potentiate neuromuscular blockade. Cimetidine decreases clearance, increases effects. Antacids may decrease absorption.

Prehospital Considerations

- IV administration: For direct IV, give each 1 mg over 1 min either undiluted or diluted in 10 mL of 5% dextrose. For intermittent infusion, further dilute in 50 mL of normal saline solution and give over 15–20 min.
- Preserve in tightly closed, light-resistant containers at 15–30C (59–86F).
- Take apical pulse and BP before administering drug.
- Withhold drug if heart rate is less than 60 bpm or systolic BP is less than 90 mm Hg.
- Careful medical history and physical examination are essential to rule out allergies, asthma, and other obstructive pulmonary disease. Propranolol can cause bronchiolar constriction even in normal subjects.
- Bradycardia is the most common adverse cardiac effect especially in patients with digitalis intoxication and Wolff-Parkinson-White syndrome.
- When propranolol is administered IV, ECG and BP must be carefully monitored. Reduction in sympathetic

stimulation caused by beta-blocking action can result in cardiac standstill.

- Adverse reactions generally occur most frequently following IV administration; however, incidence is also high following oral use in the elderly and in patients with impaired renal function. Reactions may or may not be dose related and commonly occur soon after therapy is initiated.

PROSTAGLANDIN E$_1$

Class: Vasodilator

Trade Name: Prostin VR Pediatric

Therapeutic Action/Pharmacodynamics: Prostaglandin E$_1$, also called alprostadil, is a compound derived from fatty acids that is found in several body cells. It causes vasodilation, inhibits platelet aggregation, and stimulates intestinal and uterine smooth muscle. Immediately following birth, the ductus arteriosus begins to close as blood is diverted to the pulmonary circulation. Complete closure usually occurs within one to several weeks. Some neonates and infants may suffer from one of several congenital heart diseases. Certain congenital disorders depend on a patent ductus arteriosus to prevent hypoxemia or systemic hypoperfusion. Infants with congenital heart disease may develop hypoxemia and congestive heart failure as the ductus closes. In these cases, IV administration of prostaglandin E$_1$ can keep the ductus open until a surgical repair can be made. Prostaglandin E$_1$ can also be used to "ripen" the cervix and induce labor due to its effects on uterine smooth muscle.

Emergency Uses: To maintain patency of the ductus arteriosus in infants with cyanotic congenital heart disease who are dependent on a patent ductus for life. *Adult dose:* A gel is prepared by pharmacy staff that is placed over the cervix in diaphragm. This is replaced every 2–3 hr. The patient should be monitored for fetal heart rate and contractions. *Pediatric dose:* Prostaglandin E_1 is administered IV or IO at 0.05–0.10 mcg/kg/min. Prostaglandin E_1 is used to ripen the cervix in anticipation of delivery and induces labor.

Pharmacokinetics

Absorption: Slow through vaginal mucosa. No absorption for IV dosing.

Metabolism: Approximately 68% of circulating prostaglandin E_1 is metabolized in one pass through the lungs, and the metabolites are excreted through the kidney.

Elimination: Excretion is complete within 24 hr.

Contraindications and Precautions: Prostaglandin E_1 is contraindicated in any pregnancy in which the fetus is not ready for extrauterine life. Apnea occurs in 10–12% of patients. Constant respiratory monitoring, including pulse oximetry, should be utilized.

Adverse/Side Effects: CV: Flushing, bradycardia, hypotension, tachycardia, CHF, conduction disturbances, and dysrhythmias • CNS: Seizures, hyperpyrexia, cerebral bleeding, hyperextension of the neck, hypothermia, jitteriness, and lethargy • GI: Diarrhea and gastric regurgitation • Respiratory: Apnea (usually appears in first hour and most common in infants weighing less than 2 kg at birth; bradypnea, wheezing, hypercapnea, respiratory depression, and tachypnea.

Interactions: Prostaglandin E_1 should be monitored throughout infusion and stopped immediately if worrisome symptoms develop.

Prehospital Considerations

- IV prostaglandin E_1 will be almost exclusively used in pediatric critical transport situations involving an infant with a congenital heart condition.

- The IV infusion can be prepared by placing 500 mcg in D_5W or NS.
- Smallest effective dose should be used.
- The drug should be kept refrigerated prior to use.
- Carefully monitor cardiac status, including ECG, blood pressure, pulse, and respiratory rate through course of therapy.
- Be sure to administer supplemental oxygen to infants who are dependent on a patent ductus.

RACEMIC EPINEPHRINE

Class: Sympathomimetic

Trade Names: MicroNEFRIN, Vaponephrine

Therapeutic Action/Pharmacodynamics: Racemic epinephrine is slightly different chemically from the epinephrine compounds that have been discussed previously. Compounds that differ only in their chemical arrangement are called isomers. This particular form is frequently used in children to treat croup. Racemic epinephrine stimulates both alpha- and beta-adrenergic receptors, with a slight preference for the $beta_2$ receptors in the lungs. This results in bronchodilation and a decrease in mucus secretion. It also has some effect in relieving the subglottic edema associated with croup when administered by inhalation.

Emergency Use: To relieve subglottic edema in croup (laryngotracheobronchitis). *Adult dose:* 0.25–0.75 mL of 2.25% solution in 2 mL normal saline via nebulizer. *Pediatric dose:* Same as adult.

Contraindications and Precautions: Racemic epinephrine is contraindicated in patients with a hypersensitivity to the drug, those with potential for tachydysrhythmias and hypertension, and epiglottitis.

Adverse/Side Effects: CNS: Restlessness, tremors, anxiety, nervousness, dizziness, headache • CV: Tachycardia, hypertension, palpitation, angina, dysrhythmias • Respiratory: Bronchial edema/inflammation, paradoxical bronchospasm • GI: Nausea, vomiting.

Prehospital Considerations
- Monitor vital signs prior to, during, and following administration.
- Many patients will experience rebound worsening 30–60 min after the initial treatment and the effects of the drug have worn off. For this reason, transport all patients to the hospital. Most hospitals have the policy that all children who have received racemic epinephrine will be admitted for at least 24 hr for observation.

ROCURONIUM

Class: Nondepolarizing neuromuscular blocker
Trade Name: Zemuron
Therapeutic Action/Pharmacodynamics: Rocuronium binds competitively to cholinergic receptors at the motor end plate to antagonize the action of acetylcholine. This effect is reversible with acetylcholinesterase inhibitors, such as neostigmine and edrophonium.
Emergency Uses: *Adult dose:* For rapid sequence intubation (RSI), 0.6–1.2 mg/kg will provide good intubating conditions in most patients in less than 2 min. *Pediatric dose:* For RSI, same dosing scheme as for adults.
Pharmacokinetics
Absorption: Onset in 30–60 sec; peak effect in 1–3 min; duration is 30–60 min; half-life is 14–18 min.
Contraindications and Precautions: Rocuronium is contraindicated in patients with known hypersensitivity to the drug. Use with caution in presence of cardiac disease,

lactation, children younger than 2 yr, electrolyte imbalance, dehydration, neuromuscular disease, respiratory disease, pregnancy (category C).

Adverse/Side Effects: CV: Bradycardia, tachycardia, BP changes • Respiratory: Prolonged apnea, bronchospasm, cyanosis, respiratory depression • GI: Nausea, vomiting • Skin: Rash, flushing, pruritis, urticaria.

Interactions: Pretreatment with succinylcholine, general inhalation anesthesia, lidocaine, quinidine, procainamide, beta blockers, potassium-losing diuretics, and magnesium prolongs the intensity and duration of rocuronium.

Prehospital Considerations
- Monitor vital signs closely until patient is fully recovered.
- Monitor for signs of severe allergic reaction and anaphylaxis and discontinue immediately.

SODIUM BICARBONATE (NaHCO$_3$)

Class: Electrolyte

Trade Name: Sodium bicarbonate

Therapeutic Action/Pharmacodynamics: Sodium bicarbonate is a short-acting, potent, systemic antacid. Given IV, it immediately raises the pH of blood plasma by buffering excess hydrogen ions (acidosis). In a short time, the plasma alkali reserve is increased and excess sodium and bicarbonate ions are excreted in urine, thus rendering the urine less acidic. This effect plays an important role in treating certain drug overdoses, particularly tricyclic antidepressants and barbiturates, by speeding excretion of the drug from the body. The role of sodium bicarbonate is limited in cardiac arrest. Because ventilation is an effective tool in managing respiratory acidosis, sodium bicarbonate should be considered in a prolonged cardiac arrest only after adequate airway and ventilation have been accomplished. It is considered acceptable if the arrested patient has a preexisting hyperkalemia, a preexisting bicarbonate-responsive acidosis, or a tricyclic antidepressant overdose.

Emergency Uses: To alkalinize the urine to enhance excretion of drug overdose (tricyclic antidepressants, barbiturates); to correct severe acidosis refractory to hyperventilation, known hyperkalemia. *Adult dose:* 1 mEq/kg IV; may repeat at half dose every 10 min. *Pediatric dose:* Same as adult. Can be given IO.

Pharmacokinetics
Absorption: Immediate absorption if given IV; onset is less than 15 min; duration is 1–2 hr.
Elimination: Excreted in urine within 3–4 hr.

Contraindications and Precautions: There are no absolute contraindications to using sodium bicarbonate in the above situations. When administered in large quantities, it can cause metabolic alkalosis. Always calculate the dose based on the patient's weight.

Adverse/Side Effects: Sodium bicarbonate may inhibit oxygen release secondary to a shift in oxyhemoglobin saturation. It also may produce a paradoxical acidosis that can depress cerebral and cardiac function. Sodium bicarbonate may cause extracellular alkalosis, which may reduce the concentration of ionized calcium, decrease plasma potassium, induce a left shift on the oxyhemoglobin dissociation curve, and induce malignant arrhythmias. Severe tissue damage if extravasated.

Interactions: Most catecholamines and vasopressors (dopamine, epinephrine) can be deactivated by alkaline solutions like sodium bicarbonate. When administered with calcium chloride, a precipitate may form that will clog the IV line.

Sodium Bicarbonate

Prehospital Considerations

- Infusion should be stopped immediately if extravasation occurs. Severe tissue damage has followed tissue infiltration.
- Always flush the IV line following sodium bicarbonate administration, especially in cardiac arrest.

SODIUM NITROPRUSSIDE

Class: Nitrate

Trade Names: Nipride, Nitropress

Therapeutic Action/Pharmacodynamics: Sodium nitroprusside is a potent, rapidly acting hypotensive agent with effects similar to those of the nitrates. It acts directly on vascular smooth muscle to produce peripheral vasodilation, with consequent marked lowering of arterial BP, associated with slight increase in heart rate, mild decrease in cardiac output, and moderate lowering of peripheral vascular resistance.

Emergency Use: To reduce blood pressure in an acute hypertensive crisis. *Adult dose:* 0.5–10 mcg/kg/min IV infusion. *Pediatric dose:* Same as adult.

Pharmacokinetics

Absorption: Onset is less than 1 min; peak effect in 1–5 min; duration is 1–10 min; half-life is less than 10 min after stopping infusion.

Metabolism: Rapidly converted to cyanogen in erythrocytes and tissue, which is metabolized to thiocyanate in liver.

Elimination: Excreted in urine primarily as thiocyanate.

Contraindications and Precautions: Sodium nitroprusside is contraindicated in patients with compensatory hypertension, as in atriovenous shunt or coarctation of aorta, and for control of hypertension in patients with inadequate cerebral circulation. Safe use during pregnancy (category C) is not established. Use with caution in patients with hepatic insufficiency, hypothyroidism, severe renal impairment, hyponatremia.

Adverse/Side Effects: CNS: Headache, dizziness, apprehension, restlessness, muscle twitching • CV: Profound hypotension, retrosternal discomfort, palpitation, increased or transient lowering of pulse rate, bradycardia, tachycardia, ECG changes • GI: Nausea, retching, abdominal pain • Other: Nasal stuffiness, diaphoresis • Overdosage or prolonged use (more than 48 hr): thiocyanate toxicity: profound hypotension, tinnitus, blurred vision, fatigue, metabolic acidosis, pink skin color, absence of reflexes, faint heart sounds, loss of consciousness.

Interactions: The effects of nitroprusside can be potentiated when administered with other antihypertensive agents.

Prehospital Considerations

- Solutions must be freshly prepared with D_5W and used no later than 4 hr after reconstitution.
- IV nitroprusside is diluted by dissolving 50 mg in 2–3 mL of D_5W and then further diluted in 250 mL D_5W (200 mcg/mL) or 500 mL D_5W (100 mcg/mL).
- No other drug should be added to sodium nitroprusside infusion.
- Following reconstitution, solutions usually have faint brownish tint; if solution is highly colored, do not use it. Promptly wrap container with aluminum foil or other opaque material to protect drug from light.
- Administer by infusion pump or similar device that will allow precise measurement of flow rate required to lower BP.
- Protect drug from light, heat, and moisture; store at 15–30C (59–86F) unless otherwise directed.

Sodium Nitroprusside

- Constant monitoring is required to titrate IV infusion rate to BP response.
- Adverse effects are usually relieved by slowing the IV rate or by stopping drug; they may be minimized by keeping patient supine.
- If BP begins to rise after drug infusion rate is decreased or infusion is discontinued, notify physician immediately.

SOTALOL

Classes: Beta blocker; antidysrhythmic

Trade Name: Betapace

Therapeutic Action/Pharmacodynamics: Sotalol is a nonselective beta-blocking agent with class II and class III antidysrhythmic properties. It slows the heart rate, decreases AV nodal conduction, and increases AV nodal refractoriness. Sotalol produces significant reductions in both systolic and diastolic blood pressure. It is used both orally and intravenously for ventricular and supraventricular dysrhythmias.

Emergency Use: To convert ventricular and supraventricular dysrhythmias. *Adult dose:* 1–1.5 mg/kg IV at a rate of 10 mg/min. The oral dose is 80 mg PO bid or 160 mg PO QD taken prior to meals. *Pediatric dose:* Not indicated.

Pharmacokinetics

Absorption: Slowly and completely absorbed from GI tract. Negligible first-pass metabolism. Absorption of sotalol may be reduced by food, especially milk and milk products. Peak effect in 2–3 hr; duration is 24 hr; half-life is 7–18 hr.

Distribution: Drug is hydrophilic and will enter the CSF slowly (about 10%). Crosses placental barrier. Distributed in breast milk. Not appreciably protein bound.

Metabolism: Does not undergo significant hepatic enzyme metabolism, and no active metabolites have been identified.

Elimination: Excreted by glomerular filtration in the urine with 75% of the drug excreted unchanged within 72 hr.

Contraindications and Precautions: Sotalol is contraindicated in patients with bronchial asthma, sinus bradycardia, second- and third-degree heart block, long QT syndromes, cardiogenic shock, uncontrolled CHF, chronic bronchitis, emphysema, hypersensitivity to sotalol. Use with caution in patients with CHF, electrolyte disturbances, recent MI, diabetes, sick sinus rhythms, renal impairment.

Adverse/Side Effects: CV: AV block, hypotension, aggravation of CHF (although the incidence of heart failure may be lower than for other beta blockers), life-threatening ventricular arrhythmias, including polymorphous ventricular tachycardia or *torsade de pointes*, bradycardia, dyspnea, chest pain, palpitation, bleeding (less than 2%) • CNS: Headache, fatigue, dizziness, weakness, lethargy, depression, lassitude • GI: Nausea, vomiting, diarrhea, dyspepsia, dry mouth • GU: Impotence, decreased libido • Metabolic: Hyperglycemia • Other: Visual disturbances, respiratory complaints, and rash.

Interactions: Sotalol antagonizes the effects of beta agonists. Amiodarone may lead to symptomatic bradycardia and sinus arrest. Astemizole may prolong QT interval, leading to dysrhythmias. The hypoglycemic effects of oral hypoglycemic agents may be potentiated. May cause resistance to epinephrine in anaphylactic reactions. Should be used with caution with other antidysrhythmic agents. Drug-food: absorption of sotalol may be reduced by food, especially milk and milk products.

Sotalol

Prehospital Considerations

- IV sotalol is not available in the United States.
- IV sotalol is limited by its need to be infused slowly. This may be impractical and has uncertain efficacy in emergent situations, particularly under compromised circulatory conditions.
- Smallest effective dose should be used for patients with nonallergic bronchospasms.
- Discontinuation of sotalol should not be abrupt. Dose should gradually be reduced over 1–2 wk.
- Carefully monitor cardiac status, including ECG, through course of therapy. Special caution is warranted when sotalol is used concurrently with other antidysrhythmics, digoxin, or calcium channel blockers.
- Carefully monitor patients with bronchospastic disease (e.g., bronchitis, emphysema) for inhibition of bronchodilation.
- Monitor diabetics for loss of glycemic control. Beta blockage reduces the release of endogenous insulin in response to hyperglycemia and may blunt symptoms of acute hypoglycemia (e.g., tachycardia, BP changes).

STREPTOKINASE

Class: Fibrinolytic

Trade Names: Kabikinase, Streptase

Therapeutic Action/Pharmacodynamics: Streptokinase is a derivative of the beta-hemolytic streptococci. It promotes fibrinolysis by activating the conversion of plasminogen to plasmin, the enzyme that degrades fibrin, fibrinogen, and other procoagulant proteins into soluble fragments. This fibrinolytic activity is effective both outside and within the formed thrombus/embolus. It also decreases blood and plasma viscosity and erythrocyte aggregation tendency, thus increasing perfusion of collateral blood vessels.

Emergency Uses: To reduce infarct size in acute MI by fibrinolysis. *Adult dose:* 1.5 million U IV over 1 hr. *Pediatric dose:* Not used. As a fibrinolytic for clots in deep veins (DVT) and acute pulmonary embolism. *Adult dose:* 250,000 U IV over 30 min loading dose. Maintenance dose is 100,000 U/hr for 48–72 hr. *Pediatric dose:* Not used.

Pharmacokinetics

Absorption: Onset is less than 1 hr; peak effect in 80 min; duration is 2–36 hr; half-life is 83 min.
Metabolism: Rapidly cleared from circulation by antibodies.
Elimination: Does not cross placenta, but antibodies do.

Contraindications and Precautions: Streptokinase is absolutely contraindicated in patients with active internal bleeding, suspected aortic dissection, traumatic CPR (rib fractures, pneumothorax), history of recent stroke (within 6 months), recent (within 2 months) intracranial or intraspinal surgery or trauma, intracranial tumors, uncontrolled hypertension, pregnancy, or severe allergic reactions to either anistreplase or streptokinase. Use with caution in patients over age 75 and in those with recent major surgery (within 10 days), cerebral vascular disease, recent GI or GU bleeding, recent trauma, hypertension, hemorrhagic ophthalmic conditions, and current use of oral anticoagulants.

Adverse/Side Effects: Allergic: Major (12%) (bronchospasm, periorbital swelling, angioneurotic edema, anaphylaxis); mild (urticaria, itching, headache, musculoskeletal pain, flushing, nausea, pyrexia) • Hematologic: Phlebitis, bleeding or oozing at sites of percutaneous trauma; prolonged systemic hypocoagulability; spontaneous bleeding (GU, GI, retroperitoneal); unstable blood pressure; reperfusion dysrhythmias.

Streptokinase

Interactions: Anticoagulants, NSAIDs increase the risk of bleeding; aminocaproic acid reverses the action of streptokinase.

Prehospital Considerations

- IV preparation: Streptokinase is reconstituted with 5 mL 0.9% NaCl injection (preferred) or 5 mL 5% dextrose injection. Roll or tilt vial; avoid shaking to prevent foaming or increase in flocculation. Reconstituted solution may be carefully diluted again, avoiding shaking or agitation of the solution. Slight flocculation does not interfere with drug action; discard solution with large amount of flocculi.

- Observe infusion site frequently. If phlebitis occurs, it can usually be controlled by diluting the infusion solution.

- Reconstituted solution should be stored at 2–4C (36–39F). Discard after 24 hr. Store unopened vials at 15–30C (59–86F).

- Thrombi more than 7 days old respond poorly to streptokinase therapy; therefore, IV infusion is started as soon as possible after the thrombotic event. It is most beneficial within 4 hr for AMI, up to 24 hr for PE, DVT, or arterial thrombosis.

- Spontaneous bleeding occurs about twice as often with streptokinase as with heparin. Protect patient from invasive procedures. IM injections are contraindicated. Also prevent undue manipulation during fibrinolytic therapy to prevent bruising.

- Monitor for excessive bleeding every 15 min for the first hour of therapy, every 30 min for second to eighth hour, then every 8 hr.

- Report signs of potential serious bleeding: gum bleeding, epistaxis, hematoma, spontaneous ecchymoses, oozing at catheter site, increased pulse, pain from internal bleeding. Streptokinase infusion should be interrupted, then resumed when bleeding stops.

Streptokinase

- Report promptly symptoms of a major allergic reaction; therapy will be discontinued and emergency treatment instituted. Minor symptoms (e.g., itching, nausea) respond to concurrent antihistamine or corticosteroid treatment or both without interruption of streptokinase administration.
- Check pulse frequently. Be alert to changes in cardiac rhythm, especially during intracoronary instillation. Dysrhythmias signal need to stop therapy at once.
- Monitor BP. Mild changes can be expected, but report substantial changes (greater than 25 mm Hg). Therapy may be discontinued.
- Patients who have had streptokinase previously should not receive the drug a second time because of the possibility of a severe allergic reaction.

SUCCINYLCHOLINE

Class: Depolarizing neuromuscular blocker
Trade Names: Anectine, Quelicin, Scoline (Aus), Sucostrin
Therapeutic Action/Pharmacodynamics:
Succinylcholine is a synthetic, ultra-short-acting depolarizing neuromuscular blocking agent with high affinity for acetylcholine (ACh) receptor sites. Its initial transient contractions and fasciculations are followed by sustained flaccid skeletal muscle paralysis produced by state of accommodation that develops in adjacent excitable muscle membranes. It is rapidly hydrolyzed by plasma pseudocholinesterase. It may increase vagal tone initially, particularly in children and with high doses, and subsequently produce mild sympathetic stimulation. Following IV injection, muscle paralysis begins at the eyelids and jaw, then progresses to the limbs, the abdomen, and diaphragm. There is no effect on level of consciousness.

Emergency Use: To facilitate endotracheal intubation. *Adult dose:* 1.0–1.5 mg/kg IV/IM. *Pediatric dose:* 1.0–2.0 mg/kg IV/IM.

Pharmacokinetics
Absorption: Onset in 0.5–1 min IV, 2–3 min IM. Duration is 2–3 min IV, 10–30 min IM.
Distribution: Crosses placenta in small amounts.
Metabolism: Metabolized in plasma by pseudo-cholinesterases.
Elimination: Excreted in urine.

Contraindications and Precautions: Succinylcholine is contraindicated in patients with hypersensitivity to succinylcholine, family history of malignant hyperthermia, penetrating eye injuries, or narrow-angle glaucoma. Safe use in pregnancy (category C) is not established. Use with caution in patients with severe burns or severe crush injuries as cardiac and ventricular dysrhythmias have been reported; electrolyte imbalances; renal, hepatic, pulmonary, metabolic, or cardiovascular disorders; fractures, spinal cord injury, severe liver disease, severe anemia, dehydration; collagen disorders, porphyria, intraocular surgery, glaucoma.

Adverse/Side Effects: CNS: Muscle fasciculations, profound and prolonged muscle relaxation, muscle pain • CV: Bradycardia, tachycardia, hypotension, hypertension, dysrhythmias, sinus arrest • Respiratory: Respiratory depression, bronchospasm, hypoxia, apnea • Other: Malignant hyperthermia, increased intraocular pressure, excessive salivation, enlarged salivary glands, myoglobinemia, hyperkalemia; decreased tone and motility of GI tract (large doses).

Interactions: Aminoglycosides, colistin, cyclophosphamide, cyclopropane, echothiophate iodide, halothane, lidocaine, magnesium salts, methotrimeprazine, narcotic analgesics, organophosphate insecticides, MAO inhibitors, phenothiazines, procaine, procainamide, quinidine, quinine, propranolol may prolong neuromuscular blockade. Digitalis glycosides may increase risk of cardiac dysrhythmias.

Prehospital Considerations

- Only freshly prepared solutions should be used; succinylcholine hydrolyzes rapidly with consequent loss of potency.
- IM injections are made deeply, preferably high into deltoid muscle.
- IV preparation (for prolonged paralysis): IV succinylcholine may be diluted, 1 g in 1 L of D_5W or NS, and given by intermittent or continuous infusion at a rate not to exceed 10 mg/min. A nondepolarizing agent, such as vecuronium or pancuronium, is preferred for prolonged neuromuscular blockade.
- IV administration: IV succinylcholine chloride may be given by direct IV undiluted over 10–30 sec.
- Facilities for emergency endotracheal intubation and positive pressure ventilation with oxygen should be immediately available.
- Tachyphylaxis (reduced response) may occur after repeated doses.
- Adverse effects are primarily extensions of pharmacologic actions.
- Monitor vital signs and keep airway clear of secretions.
- All resuscitation equipment should be immediately available before administering a neuromuscular blocker.

TENECTEPLASE

Class: Anticoagulant

Trade Name: TNKase

Therapeutic Action/Pharmacodynamics: Tenecteplase is a third-generation fibrinolytic agent. Its long half-life, rapid thrombolysis, and greater fibrin specificity make it an effective agent in fibrinolysis of a clot involved in a myocardial infarction.

Emergency Use: Reduction of mortality associated with acute myocardial infarction (AMI).

Adult dose:

Patient Weight (kg)	TNKase Dose (mg)	Volume TNKase to Be Administered (mL)
<60	30	6
≥60 to <70	35	7
≥70 to <80	40	8
≥80 to <90	45	9
>90	50	10

Pediatric dose: Safety in children not established.

Pharmacokinetics

Absorption: Half-life is 90–130 min.

Metabolism: Metabolized in liver.

Contraindications and Precautions: Active internal bleeding; history of CVA; intracranial or intraspinal surgery within 2 months; intracranial neoplasm; arteriovenous malformation or aneurysm; known bleeding diathesis; severe uncontrolled hypertension. Use with caution in patients with recent major surgery, previous puncture of noncompressible vessels, CVA, recent GI or GU bleeding, recent trauma; hypertension, mitral valve stenosis, acute pericarditis, bacterial endocarditis; severe liver or kidney disease; hemorrhagic ophthalmic conditions; septic thrombophlebitis or occluded, infected AV cannula; advanced age; concurrent administration of oral anticoagulants, recent administration of GP IIb/IIIa inhibitors, condition involving bleeding; pregnancy (category C), lactation. Safety and efficacy in children are not established.

Tenecteplase

Adverse/Side Effects: Hematologic: Major bleeding, hematoma, GI bleed, bleeding at puncture site, hematuria, pharyngeal, epistaxis.

Interactions: None.

Prehospital Considerations

- Avoid IM injections and unnecessary handling or invasive procedures for the first few hours after treatment.
- Monitor for signs and symptoms of bleeding. Should bleeding occur, discontinue concomitant heparin and antiplatelet therapy; notify physician.
- Monitor cardiovascular and neurologic status closely. Persons at increased risk for life-threatening cardiac events include those with a high potential for bleeding, recent surgery, severe hypertension, mitral stenosis and atrial fibrillation, anticoagulant therapy, and advanced age.
- Notify physician of the following immediately: a sudden, severe headache; any sign of bleeding; signs or symptoms of hypersensitivity.

THIAMINE

Class: Vitamin

Trade Names: Betamin (Aus), Beta-Sol (Aus), Biamine

Therapeutic Action/Pharmacodynamics: Thiamine is a water-soluble vitamin and member of the B-complex group. It functions as an essential coenzyme in carbohydrate metabolism. Thiamine is not produced by the body but must be obtained through the diet. It is required for the conversion of pyruvic acid to acetyl coenzyme A. Without thiamine, a significant amount of the energy available in glucose cannot be obtained. The brain is extremely sensitive to thiamine deficiency. Chronic alcoholic intake interferes with the absorption, intake, and use of thiamine; thus a significant number of alcoholics have thiamine deficiency. Two serious neurologic conditions, Wernicke's syndrome and Korsakoff's psychosis, can result from thiamine deficiency.

Emergency Uses: To treat coma of unknown origin, especially if alcohol is involved, and delirium tremens. *Adult dose:* 50–100 mg IV/IM. *Pediatric dose:* 10–25 mg IV/IM.

Pharmacokinetics
Distribution: Widely distributed, including into breast milk. *Elimination:* Excreted in urine.

Adverse/Side Effects: CNS: Restlessness, weakness • CV: Cardiovascular collapse • Respiratory: Pulmonary edema • Other: Feeling of warmth, urticaria, pruritus, sweating, nausea, tightness of throat, angioneurotic edema, cyanosis, GI hemorrhage, anaphylaxis • Following rapid IV administration: Slight fall in BP.

Prehospital Considerations
- Thiamine should be given prior to dextrose to facilitate its uptake if both medications are indicated.
- IV thiamine may be given by direct IV undiluted at a rate of 100 mg over 5 min. May also be added to IV solutions and infused at ordered rate.

TIROFIBAN

Classes: Anticoagulant; antiplatelet agent; glycoprotein IIb/IIIa inhibitor
Trade Name: Aggrastat
Therapeutic Action/Pharmacodynamics: Tirofiban is an antiplatelet agent that binds to the glycoprotein IIb/IIIa receptor of platelets and inhibits platelet aggregation. Its effectiveness is indicated by minimizing thrombotic events during treatment of acute coronary syndrome.

Emergency Uses: Acute coronary syndromes (unstable angina, MI). *Adult dose:* 0.4 mcg/kg/min for 30 min, followed by 0.1 mcg/kg/min. Therapy should continue through angiography and for 12–24 hr after angioplasty or atherectomy. *Pediatric dose:* Safety not established.

Pharmacokinetics

Absorption: Immediately absorbed into blood; duration is 4–8 hr after stopping infusion; half-life is 2 hours.
Distribution: 65% protein bound.
Metabolism: Minimally metabolized.
Elimination: 65% excreted in urine, 25% in feces.

Contraindications and Precautions: Active internal bleeding within 30 days; acute pericarditis; aortic dissection; concurrent use with another glycoprotein IIb/IIIa receptor inhibitor (e.g., eptifibatide, abciximab); history of aneurysm or AV malformation; history of intracranial hemorrhage or neoplasm; hypersensitivity to tirofiban; major surgery or trauma within 3 days; stroke within 30 days; history of hemorrhagic stroke; thrombocytopenia following administration of tirofiban; pregnancy (category B); lactation. Use with caution in conjunction with thrombolytic agents or drugs that cause hemolysis; hemorrhagic retinopathy; severe renal insufficiency. Safety and efficacy in children younger than 18 yr are unknown.

Adverse/Side Effects: General: Edema, swelling, pelvic pain, vasovagal reaction, leg pain • CNS: Dizziness • CV: Bradycardia, coronary artery dissection • GI: Bleeding • Hematologic: Bleeding (major bleeding), anemia, thrombocytopenia • Skin: Sweating.

Interactions: Increased risk of bleeding with anticoagulants, NSAIDs, salicylates, antiplatelet agents. Herbals such as feverfew, garlic, ginger, ginkgo, horse chestnut may increase risk of bleeding.

Tirofiban

Prehospital Considerations

- Monitor carefully for and immediately report signs and symptoms of internal or external bleeding.
- Minimize unnecessary invasive procedures and devices to reduce the risk of bleeding.

VASOPRESSIN

Classes: Hormone; vasopressor

Trade Name: Pitressin

Therapeutic Action/Pharmacodynamics: Vasopressin is a polypeptide hormone extracted from animal posterior pituitaries. It possesses pressor and antidiuretic (ADH) principles but is relatively free of oxytocic properties. Vasopressin produces concentrated urine by increasing tubular reabsorption of water (ADH activity), thus preserving up to 90% water. It may increase sodium and decrease potassium reabsorption but plays no causative role in edema formation. Small doses may produce anginal pain; large doses may precipitate MI, decrease heart rate and cardiac output, and increase pulmonary arterial pressure and BP. In unnaturally high doses (higher than those needed for antidiuretic effects), vasopressin acts as a nonadrenergic vasoconstrictor. It acts by direct stimulation of smooth muscle (V_1) receptors. It can be used as an alternative to epinephrine during CPR.

Emergency Uses: To increase peripheral vascular resistance during CPR (as an alternative to epinephrine) or after epinephrine has been used. *Adult dose:* 40 U IV (single dose only). Vasopressin is used to control bleeding from esophageal varices. It is administered by IV infusion at 0.2–0.4 U/min.

Pharmacokinetics

Absorption: Duration is 30–60 min IV infusion; half-life is 10–20 min.

Distribution: Extracellular fluid.
Metabolism: Metabolized in liver and kidneys.
Elimination: Excreted in urine.

Contraindications and Precautions: Vasopressin is contraindicated in patients with chronic nephritis accompanied by nitrogen retention; ischemic heart disease, PVCs, advanced arteriosclerosis; during first stage of labor. Use with caution in patients with epilepsy; migraine; asthma; heart failure; angina pectoris; any state in which rapid addition to extracellular fluid may be hazardous; vascular disease; preoperative and postoperative polyuric patients; renal disease; goiter with cardiac complications; and in elderly patients and children.

Adverse/Side Effects: Infrequent with low doses. Large doses: blanching of skin, abdominal cramps, nausea (almost spontaneously reversible), hypertension, bradycardia, minor arrhythmias, premature atrial contraction, heart block, peripheral vascular collapse, coronary insufficiency, MI.

Interactions: Alcohol, demeclocycline, epinephrine, heparin, lithium, phenytoin may decrease antidiuretic effects of vasopressin; guanethidine, neostigmine increase vasopressor actions; chlorpropamide, clofibrate, carbamazepine, thiazide diuretics may increase antidiuretic activity.

Prehospital Considerations
- Conclusive evidence supporting the use of vasopressin in cardiac arrest is lacking. Its use in refractory VF is class IIb (acceptable). Its use in asystole, PEA, and prolonged cardiac arrest is indeterminate (neither recommended nor forbidden).
- Vasopressin may be useful in septic shock. It is a class IIb when used when standard therapy (inotropic agents and vasoconstrictor drugs commonly used) is inadequate.

Vasopressin

- When used in vasopressor doses, as in the treatment of bleeding esophageal varices, it is common practice to administer IV nitroglycerin to help maintain mesenteric and intestinal perfusion.

VECURONIUM

Class: Nondepolarizing skeletal muscle relaxant

Trade Name: Norcuron

Therapeutic Action/Pharmacodynamics: Vecuronium is an intermediate-acting nondepolarizing skeletal muscle relaxant structurally similar to pancuronium. Unlike older neuromuscular blocking agents, it demonstrates negligible histamine release and therefore has minimal direct effect on the cardiovascular system. It is similar to atracurium in having unique metabolic and excretion pathways. In common with other drugs of this class, vecuronium inhibits neuromuscular transmission by competitive binding with acetylcholine to motor endplate receptors. It is given only after induction of general anesthesia.

Emergency Use: To facilitate endotracheal intubation. *Adult dose*: 0.08–0.10 mg/kg IV. *Pediatric dose (1 yr or older):* Same as adult.

Pharmacokinetics

Absorption: Onset is less than 1 min; peak effects in 3–5 min; duration is 25–40 min; half-life is 30–80 min.

Distribution: Well distributed to tissues and extracellular fluids; crosses placenta; distribution into breast milk unknown.

Metabolism: Rapid nonenzymatic degradation in bloodstream.

Elimination: 30–35% excreted in urine, 30–35% in bile.

Contraindications and Precautions: Vecuronium is contraindicated in patients with a hypersensitivity to the drug.

Vecuronium

Safe use during pregnancy (category C), in nursing mothers, and in neonates is not established. Use with caution in patients with severe hepatic disease; impaired acid-base or fluid/electrolyte balance; severe obesity; adrenal or neuromuscular disease (myasthenia gravis); patients with slow circulation time (cardiovascular disease, old age, edematous states); malignant hyperthermia.

Adverse/Side Effects: CNS: Skeletal muscle weakness • Respiratory: Respiratory depression • Other: Malignant hyperthermia.

Interactions: General anesthetics increase neuromuscular blockade and duration of action. Aminoglycosides, bacitracin, polymyxin B, clindamycin, lidocaine, parenteral magnesium, quinidine, quinine, trimethaphan, and verapamil increase neuromuscular blockade. Diuretics may increase or decrease neuromuscular blockade. Lithium prolongs duration of neuromuscular blockade. Narcotic analgesics increase possibility of additive respiratory depression. Succinylcholine increases onset and depth of neuromuscular blockade. Phenytoin may cause resistance to or reversal of neuromuscular blockade.

Prehospital Considerations

- Monitor vital signs at least every 15 min until stable, then every 30 min for the next 2 hr. Also monitor airway patency until assured that patient has fully recovered from drug effects. Note rate, depth, and pattern of respirations. Obese patients and patients with myasthenia gravis or other neuromuscular disease may pose ventilation problems.

- Evaluate patients for recovery from neuromuscular blocking (curare-like) effects as evidenced by ability to breathe naturally or take deep breaths and cough, to keep eyes open, and to lift head keeping mouth closed and by adequacy of hand grip strength. Notify physician if recovery is delayed.

- Note that recovery time may be delayed in patients with cardiovascular disease, edematous states, and in the elderly.
- All resuscitation equipment and supplies must be readily available before administering a neuromuscular blocker.
- Vecuronium is often used as the primary neuromuscular blocker in some EMS systems because it is nondepolarizing and does not require refrigeration.

VERAPAMIL

Class: Calcium channel blocker

Trade Names: Anpec (Aus), Calan, Cordilox (Aus), Isoptin, Novo-Veramil (Can), Verelan

Therapeutic Action/Pharmacodynamics: Verapamil inhibits calcium ion influx through slow channels into cells of myocardial and arterial smooth muscle. It dilates the coronary arteries and arterioles and inhibits coronary artery spasm; thus, myocardial oxygen delivery is increased (antianginal effect). It also decreases and slows SA and AV node conduction (antidysrhythmic effect) without effect on normal atrial action potential or intra-ventricular conduction. By vasodilation of peripheral arterioles, the drug decreases total peripheral vascular resistance and reduces arterial BP at rest. Verapamil may slightly decrease heart rate.

Emergency Uses: To convert paroxysmal supraventricular tachycardia (PSVT) refractory to adenosine; to convert atrial fibrillation and atrial flutter. *Adult dose:* 2.5–5.0 mg slow IV. May repeat at double dose in 15–30 min as needed. Do not exceed 30 mg in 30 min. *Pediatric dose:* Newborn to 1 yr: 0.1–0.2 mg/kg (not to exceed 2 mg) IV; age 1–15 yr: 0.1–0.3 mg/kg (not to exceed 5 mg) IV.

Pharmacokinetics

Absorption: Onset is 5 min; peak effect in 5–15 min; duration is 10–60 min; half-life is 2–8 hr.
Distribution: Widely distributed, including CNS; crosses placenta; present in breast milk.
Metabolism: Metabolized in liver.
Elimination: 70% excreted in urine; 16% in feces.

Contraindications and Precautions: Verapamil is contraindicated in severe hypotension (systolic less than 90 mm Hg), cardiogenic shock, cardiomegaly, digitalis toxicity, second- or third-degree AV block, Wolff-Parkinson-White syndrome including atrial flutter and fibrillation, accessory AV pathway, left ventricular dysfunction, severe congestive heart failure, sinus node disease, and sick sinus syndrome (except in patient with functioning ventricular pacemaker). Safe use during pregnancy (category C), in nursing mothers, or in children (oral) is not established. Use with caution in patients with Duchenne's muscular dystrophy; hepatic and renal impairment; MI followed by coronary occlusion or aortic stenosis.

Adverse/Side Effects: CNS: Dizziness, vertigo, headache, fatigue, sleep disturbances, depression, syncope • CV: Hypotension, CHF, bradycardia, severe tachycardia, peripheral edema, AV block • GI: Nausea, abdominal discomfort, constipation • Other: Pruritus, flushing, pulmonary edema, muscle fatigue, diaphoresis, elevated liver enzymes.

Interactions: Beta blockers increase risk of CHF, bradycardia, or heart block. Increases serum levels and toxicity of digoxin, carbamazepine, cyclosporine, lithium. Potentiates hypotensive effects of other antihypertensive agents. Verapamil effects antagonized by calcium chloride.

Verapamil

Prehospital Considerations

- IV injection: IV verapamil may be given by direct IV diluted in 5 mL of sterile water for injection at a rate of 10 mg/min.
- Inspect parenteral drug preparation before administration. Solution should be clear and colorless.
- Establish baseline data and periodically monitor BP, pulse, and hepatic and renal function.
- Transient asymptomatic hypotension may accompany IV bolus. Instruct patient to remain in recumbent position for at least 1 hr after dose is given to diminish subjective effects of hypotension.
- If IV verapamil is given concurrently with digitalis, monitor for AV block or excessive bradycardia.
- The incidence of adverse reactions is highest with IV administration, in the elderly, in patients with impaired renal function, and in patients of small stature. Drug action may be prolonged in these patients. Continuous ECG monitoring during IV administration is essential.

ZIPRASIDONE

Class: Antipsychotic

Trade Name: Geodon

Therapeutic Action/Pharmacodynamics: Unrelated to phenothiazine or butyrophenone antipsychotic agents, ziprasidone exhibits high in vitro binding affinity for dopamine, serotonin, and the alpha$_1$-adrenergic receptors. It also exhibits moderate affinity for the histamine H$_1$ receptor. Its mechanism of action is unknown; probably related to inhibition of synaptic reuptake of serotonin and norepinephrine through antagonism of dopamine and serotonin antagonism.

Emergency Uses: For treatment of acute schizophrenia, acute bipolar mania. *Adult dose:* 10-20 mg IM. *Pediatric dose:* Safety in children has not been established.

Pharmacokinetics

Absorption: Well absorbed, with 60% reaching systemic circulation; peak effects in 6–8 hr; half-life is 7 hr. *Metabolism:* Extensively metabolized in the liver. *Elimination:* 20% of metabolites excreted in urine; 66% of metabolites excreted in bile.

Contraindications and Precautions: Do not use in patients with delirium due to dementia-induced psychosis, hypersensitivity to ziprasidone; history of QT prolongation, including congenital long QT syndrome or with other drugs known to prolong the QT interval; AV block, bundle branch block, cardiac arrhythmias, congenital heart disease, recent MI or uncompensated heart failure; bradycardia, hypokalemia, or hypomagnesemia; IV administration; neuroleptic malignant syndrome and tardive dyskinesia; dehydration or hypovolemia; UV exposure and tanning beds; pregnancy (category C), lactation. Safety and efficacy in children are not established. Use with caution in patients with history of seizures, CVA, dementia, Parkinson's disease, or Alzheimer disease; known cardiovascular disease, conduction abnormalities, treatment with antihypertensive drugs; cerebrovascular disease; hepatic impairment; seizure disorder, seizures; breast cancer; risk factors for elevated core body temperature; esophageal motility disorders and risk of aspiration pneumonia; suicide potential; children older than 7 yr for use in Tourette's syndrome only.

Adverse/Side Effects: General: Asthenia, myalgia, weight gain, flu-like syndrome, face edema, chills, hypothermia; • CNS: Somnolence, akathisia, dizziness, extrapyramidal effects, dystonia, hypertonia, agitation, tremor, dyskinesias, hostility, paresthesia, confusion, vertigo, hypokinesia, hyperkinesias, abnormal gait, oculogyric crisis, hypesthesia, ataxia, amnesia, cogwheel rigidity, delirium, hypotonia, akinesia, dysarthria, withdrawal syndrome, buccoglossal syndrome, choreoathetosis, diplopia, incoordination, neuropathy • CV: Tachycardia, postural hypotension, prolonged QTc interval, hypertension • GI: Nausea, constipation, dyspepsia, diarrhea, dry mouth, anorexia, abdominal pain, vomiting • Metabolic: Hyperglycemia, diabetes mellitus • Respiratory: Rhinitis, increased cough, dyspnea • Skin: Rash, fungal dermatitis, photosensitivity • Special senses: Abnormal vision.

Interactions: Carbamazepine may decrease ziprasidone levels; ketoconazole may increase ziprasidone levels; may enhance hypotensive effects of antihypertensive agents; may antagonize effects of levodopa; increased risk of arrhythmias and heart block due to prolonged QTc interval with antiarrhythmic agents, amoxapine, arsenic trioxide, cisapride, chlorpromazine, clarithromycin, daunorubicin, diltiazem, dolasetron, doxorubicin, droperidol, erythromycin, halofantrine, indapamide, levomethadyl, local anesthetics, maprotiline, mefloquine, mesoridazine, octreotide, pentamidine, pimozide, probucol, gatifloxacin, grepafloxacin, levofloxacin, moxifloxacin, sparfloxacin, tricyclic antidepressants, tacrolimus, thioridazine, troleandomycin; additive CNS depression with sedative-hypnotics, anxiolytics, ethanol, opiate antagonists.

Prehospital Considerations

- Elderly patients with dementia-related psychosis treated with atypical antipsychotics (such as Zyprexa) are at increased risk of death and thus this class of drugs should not be used.
- Do NOT administer to anyone with a history of cardiac arrhythmias or other cardiac disease, hypokalemia,

hypomagnesemia, or prolonged QT/QTc interval, or to anyone on other drugs known to prolong the QTc interval. Withhold drug and consult physician if any of the foregoing conditions are present.

- Monitor for signs and symptoms of *torsade de pointes* (e.g., dizziness, palpitations, syncope), tardive dyskinesia especially in older adult women and with prolonged therapy, and the appearance of an unexplained rash. Withhold drug and report to physician immediately if any of these develop.
- Monitor BP lying, sitting, and standing. Report orthostatic hypotension to physician.
- Monitor cognitive status and take appropriate precautions.
- Monitor for loss of seizure control, especially with a history of seizures or dementia.

Ziprasidone

Commonly Prescribed Medications

Commonly Prescribed Medication Classes

ACE inhibitor
Prevents the conversion of angiotensin I into angiotensin II. Prescribed for hypertension and CHF.

Adrenergic antagonist
Prevents the binding of norepinephrine and epinephrine at receptor sites. Prescribed for a wide variety of conditions.

Alpha$_1$ antagonist
Blocks effects of alpha$_1$ receptors in the peripheral blood vessels. Prescribed for hypertension and BPH.

Alpha$_2$ agonist
Stimulates the alpha$_2$ receptors in the brain to inhibit presynaptic adrenergic terminals. Prescribed for hypertension.

Analgesic
Broad term referring to drugs that relieve pain.

Angiotensin II antagonist
Blocks the effects of angiotensin II at receptor sites. Prescribed for hypertension.

Anorexiant
Used to control appetite and cause weight loss.

Antialcohol
Creates unpleasant effects when alcohol is consumed. Used as a

	deterrent in chronic alcoholism.
Anti-ALS	Used to treat amyotrophic lateral sclerosis.
Antibiotic	Used to fight bacterial infection. Prescribed for a variety of infections.
Anticholinergic	Blocks acetylcholine at neuroreceptor site. Prescribed for a variety of conditions.
Anticoagulant	Interrupts the clotting cascade. Prescribed to treat deep venous thrombosis (DVT), pulmonary embolism (PE), ischemic stroke, myocardial infarction (MI).
Anticonvulsant	Broad term referring to drugs used to control seizures.
Antidepressant	Broad term referring to drugs used to treat depression.
Antidiarrheal	Inhibits bowel motility. Prescribed for diarrhea.
Antidiuretic	Inhibits diuresis.
Antidysrhythmic	Broad term referring to drugs that control and regulate the cardiac rhythm.
Antiemetic	Broad term referring to drugs used to control vomiting.

Common Medications

Antihistamine	Blocks the effects of histamine at receptor sites. H_1 blockers are prescribed for allergies. H_2 blockers are prescribed for ulcers, reflux, acid indigestion.
Antihyperlipidemic	Lowers serum cholesterol levels. Prescribed to prevent atherosclerosis.
Antihypertensive	Broad term referring to drugs that lower the blood pressure.
Antimigraine	Used to treat migraine headaches.
Antineoplastic	Kills cancer cells by a variety of mechanisms. Prescribed to treat a variety of cancers.
Antiparkinson	Increases stimulation of dopamine receptors in the brain. Prescribed to manage symptoms of Parkinson's disease.
Antiplatelet	Decreases the formation of platelet aggregates. Prescribed to prevent MI and stroke.
Antipsychotic	Broad term referring to drugs used to treat a variety of psychiatric conditions.
Antireflux	Controls esophageal reflux.

Antiseizure	Controls seizure activity in the brain.
Antituberculosis	Kills the tuberculosis bacteria. Prescribed for suspected and confirmed tuberculosis.
Antitussive	Suppresses the cough reflex mechanism. Prescribed for cough.
Antiulcer	Reduces the secretion of acids. Prescribed for ulcers.
Antivertigo	Broad term referring to drugs used to control vertigo and motion sickness.
Antiviral	Treats viruses by a variety of mechanisms. Prescribed for a variety of viral infections, particularly HIV.
Anxiolytic	Alleviates anxiety.
Barbiturate	Causes sedative-hypnotic effect. Prescribed for seizures, anxiety.
Benzodiazepine	Causes sedative-hypnotic effect. Prescribed for seizures, anxiety, muscle relaxant.
Beta blocker	Blocks the effects of epinephrine at beta receptor sites. Prescribed for angina, hypertension, tachydysrhythmias.

Common Medications

Bronchodilator	Dilates the bronchiole smooth muscles by a variety of mechanisms.
Calcium channel blocker	Inhibits the influx of calcium into the cell. Prescribed for angina, hypertension, tachydysrhythmias.
Cardiac glycoside	Lowers heart rate while increasing the force of contraction. Prescribed for tachydysrhythmias, congestive heart failure.
Cholinergic	Stimulates binding of acetylcholine with muscarinic receptors, particularly in bladder and GI tract. Prescribed to increase urination and peristalsis.
Cholinesterase inhibitor	Prolongs the effects of acetylcholine by inhibiting its breakdown. Prescribed for myasthenia gravis, some types of poi-soning, and glaucoma.
CNS stimulant	Increases CNS depolarization, prescribed for fatigue, narcolepsy, obesity, attention deficit hyperactivity disorder (ADHD), drowsiness.

Decongestant	Relieves upper respiratory tract congestion.
Digestant	Mimics the pancreatic enzymes and aids in digestion of food.
Diuretic	Stimulates the kidneys to produce more urine. Prescribed for hypertension and congestive heart failure.
Estrogen hormone	Replaces estrogen in postmenopausal women.
Glucocorticoid	Reduces the inflammatory process. Prescribed for asthma and other causes of inflammation.
Hormone	Simulates the action of various glands. Prescribed for a variety of conditions that affect the endocrine system.
Hypnotic	Induces sleep.
Immunosuppressant	Used with transplant surgery to decrease incidence of rejection. Also to treat some cancers.
Infertility agent	Promotes the maturation of ovarian follicles. Prescribed to treat infertility.

Insulin preparation	Facilitates the diffusion of glucose into the cells. Prescribed for insulin-dependent diabetes mellitus.
Laxative	Alters the consistency of stool. Prescribed for constipation.
Leukotriene antagonist	Blocks the effects of leukotrienes at receptor sites. Prescribed for asthma.
MAO inhibitor	Inhibits breakdown of monamine oxidase (MAO). Prescribed for depression.
Mast cell stabilizer	Prevents mast cells from secreting histamine.
Methylxanthine	Bronchodilates by inhibiting the breakdown of beta agonists. Prescribed for asthma.
Mood stabilizer	Prescribed for bipolar disorder (manic-depressive).
Mucolytic	Decreases the viscosity of respiratory secretions. Prescribed for upper respiratory infection, pneumonia, cystic fibrosis.
Narcotic analgesic	Contains opium or its derivative. Prescribed for moderate or severe pain relief.

Nitrate	Causes vasodilation. Prescribed for angina, congestive heart failure.
NSAID	Nonsteroidal anti-inflammatory drug; prescribed for pain, fever, inflammation, arthritis.
Oral hypoglycemic	Some stimulate the pancreas to produce insulin. Others alter the absorption of glucose from the GI tract. Prescribed for non-insulin-dependent diabetes mellitus.
Phenothiazine	Antipsychotic medications that block dopamine receptors in the brain; prescribed for schizophrenia, depression, bipolar disorder, and nausea.
Progestin hormone	Replaces progesterone in postmenopausal women. Prescribed as oral contraceptive and to treat amenorrhea, endometriosis, and uterine bleeding.
Psychotherapeutic	Broad term referring to drugs used to treat a variety of psychiatric conditions.

Common Medications

Skeletal muscle relaxant	Blocks the release of calcium from sarcoplasmic reticulum. Prescribed for muscle spasms.
SSRI	Selective serotonin reuptake inhibitor. Blocks reuptake of serotonin. Prescribed for depression and as an antipsychotic.
Stool softener	Alters the consistency of stool. Used as a laxative.
Thyroid hormone	Synthetic replica of the natural thyroid hormone.
Tricyclic antidepressant	Blocks reuptake of norepinephrine and serotonin. Prescribed for depression.
Uricosuric	Used to treat gout.
Vasodilator	Dilates the blood vessels.

List of Commonly Prescribed Medications Following is a list of commonly prescribed medications and their class. If additional information is required concerning a drug, consult the *Physician's Desk Reference* or a similar source. In the left column, trade names are capitalized, and generic names are in lower case.

acarbose	Oral hypoglycemic
Accolate	Leukotriene antagonist
Accupril	ACE inhibitor
acebutolol	Beta blocker
Aceon	ACE inhibitor
acetaminophen	Analgesic
Acetazolam	Diuretic
acetazolamide	Diuretic
acetohexamide	Oral hypoglycemic
acetylcysteine	Mucolytic
Achro-mycin	Antibiotic
Actidil	Antihistamine
Actron	NSAID
Acular	NSAID
acycloguanosine	Antiviral agent
acyclovir	Antiviral agent
Adalat	Calcium channel blocker
Adapin	Tricyclic antidepressant
Aeroseb-Dex	Glucocorticoid
Aerosporin	Antibiotic
Agrylin	Antiplatelet
Airbron	Mucolytic
Akineton	Anticholinergic (antiparkinson)
Alazine	Antihypertensive
Albamycin	Antibiotic
albendazole	Antibiotic
Albenza	Antibiotic

albuterol	Adrenergic bronchodilator
Aclovate	Glucocorticoid
alcometasone	Glucocorticoid
Aldactone	Diuretic
Aldomet	Antihypertensive
Aleve	NSAID
Alkeran	Antineoplastic
Allegra	Antihistamine
Alloprin	Uricosuric (antigout)
allopurinol	Uricosuric (antigout)
Alomide	Mast cell stabilizer
Alora	Estrogen hormone
alprazolam	Benzodiazepine
Altace	ACE inhibitor
Alupent	Adrenergic bronchodilator
Alurate	Barbiturate
amantadine	Anticholinergic (antiparkinson); antiviral agent
Amaryl	Oral hypoglycemic
ambenonium	Cholinesterase inhibitor
Ambien	Anxiolytic
Amcill	Antibiotic
Amen	Progesterone hormone
Amerge	Antimigraine
Amethopterin	Antineoplastic
amiloride	Diuretic
aminogluthimide	Antineoplastic
Amitril	Tricyclic antidepressant
amitriptyline	Tricyclic antidepressant
amlodipine	Calcium channel blocker
amobarbital	Barbiturate

amoxapine	Tricyclic antidepressant
amoxicillin	Antibiotic
Amoxil	Antibiotic
amphetamine	CNS stimulant
ampicillin	Antibiotic
Ampicin	Antibiotic
Amytal	Barbiturate
Anafranil	Tricyclic antidepressant
anagrelide hydrochloride	Antiplatelet
anastrozole	Antineoplastic
Ancobon	Antibiotic
Ancotil	Antibiotic
Andostatin	Antidiarrheal
Ansaid	NSAID
Ansamycin	Antituberculosis
Anspor	Antibiotic
Antabuse	Antialcohol
Antazone	Uricosuric (antigout)
Antivert	Antiemetic
Antrizine	Antiemetic
Anturan	Uricosuric (antigout)
Aparkane	Anticholinergic (antiparkinson)
Apo-Amoxil	Antibiotic
Apo-Pen	Antibiotic
Apresoline	Antihypertensive
aprobarbital	Barbiturate
Aquachloral Supprettes	Anxiolytic
Aquatag	Diuretic
Aquatensen	Diuretic
Aricept	Cholinesterase inhibitor
Aristocort	Glucocorticoid
Armidex	Antineoplastic
Armour Thyroid	Thyroid hormone

Arrestin	Antiemetic
Artane	Anticholinergic (antiparkinson)
Artha	NSAID
Arthropan	NSAID
Asendin	Tricyclic antidepressant
Atabrine	Antibiotic
Atacand	Angiotensin II blocker
Atarax	Antihistamine
atenolol	Beta blocker
Ativan	Benzodiazepine
Atolone	Glucocorticoid
Atorvastatin	Antihyperlipidemic
Atromid	Antihyperlipidemic
Atrovent	Anticholinergic bronchodilator
Avapro	Angiotensin II blocker
Aventyl	Tricyclic antidepressant
Avlosulfon	Antibiotic
Axid	Antiulcer
Azactam	Antibiotic
azatadine	Antihistamine
azathioprine	Immunosuppressant
azithromycin	Antibiotic
aztreonam	Antibiotic
bacampicillin	Antibiotic
baclofen	Skeletal muscle relaxant
Bactocill	Antibiotic
Bactrim	Antibiotic
Banflex	Skeletal muscle relaxant
Barbased	Barbiturate
Baychol	Antihyperlipidemic
beclomethasone	Glucocorticoid
Beclovent	Glucocorticoid

Beconase	Glucocorticoid
Benadryl	Antihistamine
benazepril	ACE inhibitor
bendroflumethiazide	Diuretic
Benemid	Uricosuric (antigout)
Bensylate	Anticholinergic (antiparkinson)
Bentyl	Antispasmodic
Benuryl	Uricosuric (antigout)
benzonatate	Antitussive
benzphetamine	CNS stimulant
benzthiazide	Diuretic
benztropine	Anticholinergic (antiparkinson)
bepridil	Calcium channel blocker
Betaloc	Beta blocker
Betapace	Beta blocker
Betapen	Antibiotic
bethanechol	Cholinergic
Betimol	Beta blocker
Biaxin	Antibiotic
biperiden	Anticholinergic (antiparkinson)
Bishydroxycoumarin	Anticoagulant
bisoprolol	Beta blocker
bitolterol	Adrenergic bronchodilator
Blocadren	Beta blocker
Bonamine	Antiemetic
Bonine	Antiemetic
Brethaire	Adrenergic bronchodilator
Brethine	Adrenergic bronchodilator

Bricanyl	Adrenergic bronchodilator
Bromphen	Antihistamine
brompheniramine	Antihistamine
Bronkodyl	Methylxanthine bronchodilator
Bronkometer	Adrenergic bronchodilator
Bronkosol	Adrenergic bronchodilator
Bucladin	Antivertigo
buclizine	Antivertigo
budesonide	Glucocorticoid
bumetanide	Diuretic
Bumex	Diuretic
bupropion	Antidepressant
Buspar	Anxiolytic
buspirone	Anxiolytic
busulfan	Antineoplastic
butabarbital	Barbiturate
Butalan	Barbiturate
Butisol	Barbiturate
Calan	Calcium channel blocker
candesartan	Angiotensin II antagonist
capecitabine	Antineoplastic
Capoten	ACE inhibitor
captopril	ACE inhibitor
Carafate	Antiulcer
carbamazepine	Anticonvulsant
Carbatrol	Anticonvulsant
carbenicillin	Antibiotic
Carbex	MAO inhibitor
carbidopa	Anticholinergic (antiparkinson)

Carbolith	Mood stabilizer
Cardene	Calcium channel blocker
Cardioquin	Antidysrhythmic
Cardizem	Calcium channel blocker
Cardura	Alpha$_1$ blocker
carisoprodol	Skeletal muscle relaxant
carteolol	Beta blocker
Cartrol	Beta blocker
carvedilol	Antihypertensive
Catapres	Alpha$_2$ agonist
Ceclor	Antibiotic
Cedax	Antibiotic
cefaclor	Antibiotic
cefadroxil	Antibiotic
Cefanex	Antibiotic
cefdinir	Antibiotic
cefixime	Antibiotic
cefpodoxime	Antibiotic
cefproxil	Antibiotic
ceftibuten	Antibiotic
cefuroxime	Antibiotic
Cefzil	Antibiotic
Celebrex	NSAID
celecoxib	NSAID
Celexa	SSRI antidepressant
Celontin	Anticonvulsant
cephalexin	Antibiotic
cephradine	Antibiotic
Cephulac	Laxative
Ceporex	Antibiotic
Cerespan	Vasodilator
cerivastatin	Antihyperlipidemic
Cesamet	Antiemetic

Cetirizine	Antihistamine
Chibroxin	Antibiotic
chloral hydrate	Anxiolytic
chlorambucil	Antineoplastic
chlordiazepoxide	Benzodiazepine
Chloronase	Oral hypoglycemic
chlorothiazide	Diuretic
Chlorpromanyl	Phenothiazine
chlorpromazine	Phenothiazine
chlorpropamide	Oral hypoglycemic
chlorprothixene	Phenothiazine
chlorthalidone	Diuretic
chlortrianisene	Estrogen hormone
chlorzoxazone	Skeletal muscle relaxant
Choledyl	Methylxanthine bronchodilator
Cholestabyl	Antihyperlipidemic
cholestyramine	Antihyperlipidemic
choline salicylate	NSAID
Choloxin	Antihyperlipidemic
Cholybar	Antihyperlipidemic
Chronulac	Laxative
Cinobac	Antibiotic
cinoxacin	Antibiotic
Cipro	Antibiotic
ciprofloaxin	Antibiotic
cisapride	Antireflux
citalopram	SSRI antidepressant
Claripex	Antihyperlipidemic
clarithromycin	Antibiotic
Claritin	Antihistamine
Cleocin	Antibiotic
Climara	Estrogen hormone
clindamycin	Antibiotic
Clinoril	NSAID

clofibrate	Infertility agent
Clomid	Infertility agent
clomiphene	Antihyperlipidemic
clomipramine	Tricyclic antidepressant
clonazepam	Benzodiazepine
clonidine	Alpha$_2$ agonist
Clopra	Cholinergic (antiemetic)
clorazepate	Benzodiazepine
cloxacillin	Antibiotic
Clox-apen	Antibiotic
Cloxilean	Antibiotic
clozapine	Psychotherapeutic
Clozaril	Psychotherapeutic
codeine	Narcotic analgesic
Codimal	Antihistamine
Cogentin	Anticholinergic (antiparkinson)
Cognex	Cholinesterase inhibitor
Colace	Stool softener
colchicine	Uricosuric (antigout)
Colestid	Antihyperlipidemic
colestipol	Antihyperlipidemic
colistimethate	Antihyperlipidemic
Coly-Mycin	Antibiotic
Compazine	Phenothiazine
Conjec	Antihistamine
Cophene	Antihistamine
Coreg	Antihypertensive
Corgard	Beta blocker
Coronex	Nitrate
cortisone	Glucocorticoid
Cortistan	Glucocorticoid
Cortone	Glucocorticoid
Cotazym	Digestant

Coumadin	Anticoagulant
Cozaar	Angiotensin II blocker
Crinone	Progesterone hormone
Crixivan	Antiviral agent
cromolyn sodium	Mast cell stabilizer
Cronetal	Antialcohol
cyclizine	Antiemetic
cyclobenzaprine	Skeletal muscle relaxant
cycloserine	Antituberculosis
cyclosporine	Immunosuppressant
Cycoflex	Skeletal muscle relaxant
Cycrin	Progesterone hormone
Cylert	CNS stimulant
cyproheptadine	Antihistamine
Cytadren	Antineoplastic
Cytomel	Thyroid hormone
Cytotec	Antiulcer
Dalacin	Antibiotic
Dalmane	Benzodiazepine
Dantrium	Skeletal muscle relaxant
dantrolene	Skeletal muscle relaxant
dapsone	Antibiotic
Darvon	Narcotic analgesic
Datril	Analgesic
DDAVP	Antidiuretic
Decaderm	Glucocorticoid
Decadron	Glucocorticoid
Decaspray	Glucocorticoid
Declomycin	Antibiotic
Dehist	Antihistamine
delavirdine	Antiviral agent
Deltasone	Glucocorticoid
Demadex	Diuretic
demeclocycline	Antibiotic
Demerol	Narcotic analgesic

Denavir	Antiviral agent
Depacon	Anticonvulsant
Depakene	Anticonvulsant
Depakote	Anticonvulsant
Deponit	Nitrate
Depo-Provera	Progesterone hormone
Deronil	Glucocorticoid
desipramine	Tricyclic antidepressant
desmopressin	Antidiuretic hormone
Desoxyephedrine	CNS stimulant
Desoxyn	CNS stimulant
Desyrel	Antidepressant
Detrol	Anticholinergic
Dexameth	Glucocorticoid
dexamethasone	Glucocorticoid
Dexampex	CNS stimulant
Dexasone	Glucocorticoid
Dexchlor	Antihistamine
dexchlorpheniramine	Antihistamine
Dexedrine	CNS stimulant
Dexone	Glucocorticoid
dextroamphetamine	CNS stimulant
dextrothyroxine	Antihyperlipidemic
DGSS	Stool softener
DiaBeta	Oral hypoglycemic
Diabinese	Oral hypoglycemic
Diachlor	Diuretic
Diamox	Diuretic
Diapil	Antidiuretic
Diaqua	Diuretic
diazepam	Benzodiazepine
Dibenzyline	Alpha$_1$ blocker
diclofenac	NSAID
dicloxacillin	Antibiotic
dicumarol	Anticoagulant

dicyclomine	Anticholinergic; antispasmodic
didanosine	Antiviral agent
Didrex	CNS stimulant
diethylproprion	Anorexiant
Diflucan	Antibiotic
diflunisal	NSAID
digoxin	Cardiac glycoside
Dilacor	Calcium channel blocker
Dilantin	Anticonvulsant
Dilatrate	Nitrate
Dilaudid	Narcotic analgesic
Dilor	Methylxanthine bronchodilator
diltiazem	Calcium channel blocker
Dimelor	Oral hypoglycemic
dimenhydrinate	Antihistamine
Dimetane	Antihistamine
Dinate	Antihistamine
Dio-Sul	Stool softener
Diovan	Angiotensin II antagonist
Dipentum	Anti-inflammatory
diphenhydramine	Antihistamine
diphenidol	Antivertigo
dirithromycin	Antibiotic
Disalcid	NSAID
Disodium Cromoglycate	Mast cell stabilizer
Disonate	Stool softener
disopyramide	Antidysrhythmic
disulfiram	Antialcohol agent
Ditropan	Anticholinergic
Diucardin	Diuretic
Diulo	Diuretic

Diurese	Diuretic
Diuril	Diuretic
Dixaril	Alpha$_2$ agonist
Dizmiss	Antiemetic
docusate	Stool softener
Dolobid	NSAID
Dolophine	Narcotic analgesic
Dommanate	Antihistamine
donepezil	Cholinesterase inhibitor
Dopamet	Antihypertensive
Dopar	Anticholinergic (antiparkinson)
Doral	Benzodiazepine
Doriglute	Barbiturate
dornase alpha	Mucolytic
Doryx	Antibiotic
doxazosin	Alpha$_1$ blocker
doxepin	Tricyclic antidepressant
Doxy	Antibiotic
Doxychel	Antibiotic
doxycycline	Antibiotic
Dramamine	Antihistamine
Dramanate	Antihistamine
Dramilin	Antihistamine
Dramocen	Antihistamine
droperidol	Antiemetic
DSCG	Mast cell stabilizer
Duosol	Stool softener
Duotrate	Nitrate
Duraclon	Alpha$_2$ agonist
Duralith	Mood stabilizer
Durapam	Benzodiazepine
Duraquin	Antidysrhythmic
Duretic	Diuretic
Duricef	Antibiotic

Duvoid	Cholinergic
Dycill	Antibiotic
Dyflex	Methylxanthine bronchodilator
Dyl-line	Methylxanthine bronchodilator
Dymenate	Antihistamine
Dynabac	Antibiotic
Dynacirc	Calcium channel blocker
Dynapen	Antibiotic
dyphylline	Methylxanthine bronchodilator
Dyrenium	Diuretic
Edecrin	Diuretic
Efavirenz	Antiviral agent
Efedron	Decongestant
Effexor	SSRI antidepressant
Elavil	Tricyclic antidepressant
Eldepryl	MAO inhibitor
Elixophyllin	Methylxanthine bronchodilator
Eltroxin	Thyroid hormone
Emcyt	Antineoplastic
Emex	Cholinergic
Emitrip	Tricyclic antidepressant
E-Mycin	Antibiotic
enalapril	ACE inhibitor
Endep	Tricyclic antidepressant
Enduron	Diuretic
Enovil	Tricyclic antidepressant
enoxacin	Antibiotic
ephedrine	Decongestant
Epitol	Anticonvulsant
Epivir	Antiviral agent
Equanil	Anxiolytic

Erythrocin	Antibiotic
erythromycin	Antibiotic
Esidrix	Diuretic
Eskalith	Mood stabilizer
estazolam	Benzodiazepine
Estinyl	Estrogen hormone
Estrace	Estrogen hormone
Estraderm	Estrogen hormone
estradiol	Estrogen hormone
estramustine	Antineoplastic
Estring	Estrogen hormone
estrogens	Estrogen hormone
estropipate	Estrogen hormone
ethacrynic acid	Diuretic
ethambutol	Antituberculosis agent
Ethaquin	Vasodilator
Ethatab	Vasodilator
ethaverine	Vasodilator
ethchlorvynol	Barbiturate
ethinyl estradiol	Estrogen hormone
ethionamide	Antituberculosis agent
Ethmozine	Antidysrhythmic
Ethon	Diuretic
ethosuximide	Anticonvulsant
Etibi	Antituberculosis
etodolac	NSAID
Euglucon	Oral hypoglycemic
Eulexin	Antineoplastic
Euthroid	Thyroid hormone
Evista	Estrogen hormone
Exna	Diuretic
famciclovir	Antiviral agent
Famvir	Antiviral agent
Fareston	Antineoplastic
felbamate	Anticonvulsant

Felbatol	Anticonvulsant
Feldene	NSAID
felodipine	Calcium channel blocker
Femara	Antineoplastic
Feminone	Estrogen hormone
Fempatch	Estrogen hormone
fenofibrate	Antihyperlipidemic
fexofenadine	Antihistamine
Fivent	Mast cell stabilizer
Flagyl	Antibiotic
flavoxate	Anticholinergic
flecainide	Antidysrhythmic
Flexeril	Skeletal muscle relaxant
Flexon	Skeletal muscle relaxant
Flomax	Alpha$_1$ blocker
Florinef	Glucocorticoid
Floxin	Antibiotic
fluconazole	Antibiotic
flucytosine	Antibiotic
fludrocortisone	Glucocorticoid
Flumadine	Antiviral agent
fluoxetine	SSRI antidepressant
fluphenazine	Phenothiazine
flurazepam	Benzodiazepine
flurbiprofen	NSAID
Flutamide	Antineoplastic
fluvastatin	Antihyperlipidemic
fluvoxamine	SSRI antidepressant
Fortovase	Antiviral agent
fosfomycin	Antibiotic
fosinopril	ACE inhibitor
Fumide	Diuretic
Furadantin	Antibiotic
Furalan	Antibiotic
Furanite	Antibiotic

Common Medications

furazolidone	Antibiotic
Furomide	Diuretic
furosemide	Diuretic
Furoxone	Antibiotic
Gabapentin	Anticonvulsant
Gabitril Filmtabs	Anticonvulsant
Gantanol	Antibiotic
Gantrisin	Antibiotic
gemfibrozil	Antihyperlipidemic
Genabid	Vasodilator
Geocillin	Antibiotic
Geopen	Antibiotic
glimepiride	Oral hypoglycemic
glipizide	Oral hypoglycemic
Glucamide	Oral hypoglycemic
Glucophage	Oral hypoglycemic
Glucotrol	Oral hypoglycemic
glutethimide	Barbiturate
glyburide	Oral hypoglycemic
glycopyrrolate	Antiulcer
Glynase	Oral hypoglycemic
Gravol	Antihistamine
grepafloxacin	Antibiotic
guanabenz	Antihypertensive
guandrel	Antihypertensive
guanethidine	Antihypertensive
guanfacine	Antihypertensive
halazepam	Benzodiazepine
Halcion	Benzodiazepine
Haldol	Antipsychotic
Haldrone	Glucocorticoid
haloperidol	Antipsychotic
haloprogin	Antibiotic
Halotex	Antibiotic
HCTZ	Diuretic

Hexadrol	Glucocorticoid
Hexalen	Antineoplastic
hexamethylamine	Antineoplastic
Hiprex	Antibiotic
Histantil	Phenothiazine
Hivid	Antiviral agent
Honval	Estrogen hormone
Humalog	Insulin preparation
Humatin	Antibiotic
Humulin	Insulin preparation
Hycodan	Narcotic analgesic
hydralazine	Antihypertensive
Hydrate	Antihistamine
Hydrea	Antineoplastic
Hydrex	Diuretic
hydrochlorothiazide	Diuretic
hydrocodone	Narcotic analgesic
HydroDiuril	Diuretic
hydroflumethiazide	Diuretic
hydromorphone	Narcotic analgesic
hydroxyurea	Antineoplastic
hydroxyzine	Antihistamine
Hygroton	Diuretic
Hylidone	Diuretic
Hylorel	Antihypertensive
Hyoscine	Anticholinergic (antiparkinson)
Hy-Pam	Antihistamine
Hytrin	Alpha$_1$ blocker
Hyzine-50	Antihistamine
Iletin	Insulin preparation
Ilotycin	Antibiotic
Ilozyme	Digestant
Imdur	Nitrate
imipramine	Tricyclic antidepressant

Imitrex	Antimigraine
Imodium	Antidiarrheal
Impril	Tricyclic antidepressant
Imuran	Immunosuppressant
Inapsine	Antiemetic
Indameth	NSAID
indapamide	Diuretic
Inderal	Beta blocker
indinavir	Antiviral agent
Indocid	NSAID
Indocin	NSAID
indomethacin	NSAID
insulin	Insulin preparation
Intal	Mast cell stabilizer
Inversine	Antihypertensive
Invirase	Protease inhibitor
ipratroprium	Anticholinergic bronchodilator
irbesartan	Angiotensin II blocker
Ismelin	Antihypertensive
Ismo	Nitrate
Isobec	Barbiturate
Iso-Bid	Nitrate
isocarboxazid	MAO inhibitor
isoetharine	Adrenergic bronchodilator
isoproterenol	Adrenergic bronchodilator
Isoptin	Calcium channel blocker
Isordil	Nitrate
isosorbide	Nitrate
Isotrate	Nitrate
Isovex	Vasodilator
isoxuprine	Vasodilator
isradipine	Calcium channel blocker

itraconazole	Antibiotic
Janimine	Tricyclic antidepressant
kanamycin	Antibiotic
Kantrex	Antibiotic
Keflet	Antibiotic
Keflex	Antibiotic
Keftab	Antibiotic
Kefurox	Antibiotic
Kemadrin	Anticholinergic (antiparkinson)
Kenacort	Glucocorticoid
ketoconazole	Antibiotic
ketoprofen	NSAID
ketorolac	NSAID
Klonopin	Benzodiazepine
Kredex	Antihypertensive
labetolol	Beta blocker
lactulose	Laxative
Lamictal	Anticonvulsant
lamotrigine	Anticonvulsant
Lanophyllin	Methylxanthine bronchodilator
Lanoxicaps	Cardiac glycoside
Lanoxin	Cardiac glycoside
lansoprazole	Antiulcer
Largactil	Phenothiazine
Larodopa	Anticholinergic (antiparkinson)
Larotid	Antibiotic
Lasix	Diuretic
Laxinate	Stool softener
Ledercillin	Antibiotic
Lente	Insulin preparation
Lescol	Antihyperlipidemic
letrozole	Antineoplastic

Leukeran	Antineoplastic
Leutrol	Leukotriene antagonist
Levaquin	Antibiotic
Levate	Tricyclic antidepressant
Levatol	Beta blocker
levodopa	Anticholinergic (antiparkinson)
Levo-Dromoran	Narcotic analgesic
levofloxacin	Antibiotic
levomethadyl	Narcotic analgesic
levonorgestrel	Progesterone hormone
Levoprome	Phenothiazine
levorphanol	Narcotic analgesic
Levo-throid	Thyroid hormone
levothyroxine	Thyroid hormone
Levoxyl	Thyroid hormone
Libritabs	Benzodiazepine
Librium	Benzodiazepine
Lincocin	Antibiotic
lincomycin	Antibiotic
Liorsen	Skeletal muscle relaxant
liothyronine	Thyroid hormone
liotrix	Thyroid hormone
Lipitor	Antihyperlipidemic
Lipoxide	Benzodiazepine
lisinopril	ACE inhibitor
Lithane	Mood stabilizer
lithium	Mood stabilizer
Lithobid	Mood stabilizer
Lithonate	Mood stabilizer
Lithotabs	Mood stabilizer
Lodine	NSAID
Lodosyn	Anticholinergic (antiparkinson)
lodoxamide	Mast cell stabilizer

lomefloxacin	Antibiotic
lomustine	Antineoplastic
Loniten	Vasodilator
loperamide	Antidiarrheal
Lopid	Antihyperlipidemic
Lopressor	Beta blocker
Lopurin	Uricosuric (antigout)
Lorabid	Antibiotic
loracarbef	Antibiotic
loratadine	Antihistamine
lorazepam	Benzodiazepine
losartan	Angiotensin II blocker
Losec	Antiulcer
Lotensin	ACE inhibitor
lovastatin	Antihyperlipidemic
loxapine	Antipsychotic
Loxitane	Antipsychotic
Lozide	Diuretic
Lozol	Diuretic
Ludiomil	Antidepressant
Lufyllin	Methylxanthine bronchodilator
Luminal	Barbiturate
Luramide	Diuretic
Luvox	SSRI antidepressant
lypressin	Antidiuretic hormone
Lysodren	Antineoplastic
maprotiline	Antidepressant
Marazide	Diuretic
Marbaxin	Skeletal muscle relaxant
Marezine	Antiemetic
Marmine	Antihistamine
Marplan	MAO inhibitor antidepressant
Marzine	Antiemetic

Mavik	ACE inhibitor
Maxair	Adrenergic bronchodilator
Maxalt	Antimigraine
Maxaquin	Antibiotic
Maxeran	Cholinergic
Maxidex	Glucocorticoid
Maxolon	Cholinergic
Mazanor	CNS stimulant
Mazepine	Anticonvulsant
mazindol	CNS stimulant
Mebaral	Barbiturate
mecamylamine	Antihypertensive
mecaptopurine	Antineoplastic
meclizine	Antiemetic
Meclofen	NSAID
meclofenamate	NSAID
Meclomen	NSAID
Medihaler-Iso	Adrenergic bronchodilator
Medilium	Benzodiazepine
Medrol	Glucocorticoid
medroxyprogesterone	Progesterone hormone
mefenamic	NSAID
Megace	Antineoplastic
megestrol	Antineoplastic
Mellaril	Phenothiazine
melphalen	Antineoplastic
Menorest	Estrogen hormone
Menotropins	Infertility drug
meperidine	Narcotic analgesic
mephenytoin	Anticonvulsant
mephobarbital	Barbiturate
meprobamate	Anxiolytic
Meprospan	Anxiolytic

Meravil	Tricyclic antidepressant
Meridia	Appetite suppressant
Mesantoin	Anticonvulsant
mesoridazine	Phenothiazine
Metahydrin	Diuretic
Metaprel	Adrenergic bronchodilator
metaproterenol	Adrenergic bronchodilator
metformin	Oral hypoglycemic agent
methadone	Narcotic analgesic
methenamine	Antibiotic
methimazole	Antithyroid agent
methocarbamol	Skeletal muscle relaxant
methotrexate	Antineoplastic
methotrimeprazine	Phenothiazine
methscopolamine	Anticholinergic
methsuximide	Anticonvulsant
methyclothiazide	Diuretic
methyldopa	Antihypertensive
methylphenidate	CNS stimulant
Methylphenobarbital	Barbiturate
methylprednisolone	Glucocorticoid
methyprylon	Hypnotic
methysergide	Antimigraine
Metizol	Antibiotic
metoclopramide	Cholinergic
metolazone	Diuretic
metoprolol	Beta blocker
Metrodin	Infertility agent
metronidazole	Antibiotic
Mevacor	Antihyperlipidemic
Mevinolin	Antihyperlipidemic
Mexate	Antineoplastic
mexiletine	Antidysrhythmic

Mexitil	Antidysrhythmic
Mezlin	Antibiotic
mezlocillin	Antibiotic
Micronase	Oral hypoglycemic
Micronor	Progesterone hormone
Midamor	Diuretic
midodrine	Alpha$_1$ agonist
Miltown	Anxiolytic
Minipress	Alpha$_1$ blocker
Minitran	Nitrate
Minocin	Antibiotic
minocycline	Antibiotic
minoxidil	Vasodilator
Mirapex	Anticholinergic (antiparkinson)
mirtazapine	Antidepressant
misoprostol	Antiulcer
mitotane	Antineoplastic
Moban	Phenothiazine
Mobenol	Oral hypoglycemic
Modane Soft	Stool softener
moexipril	ACE inhibitor
molindone	Phenothiazine
Monitan	Beta blocker
Mono-Gesic	NSAID
Mono-ket	Nitrate
Monopril	ACE inhibitor
montelukast	Leukotriene blocker
Monurol	Antibiotic
moricizine	Antidysrhythmic
Mucomyst	Mucolytic
Mucosol	Mucolytic
Murocoll	Anticholinergic (antiparkinson)

Myambutol	Antituberculosis
Mycifradin	Antibiotic
Myciguent	Antibiotic
Mycobutin	Antituberculosis
Mycostatin	Antibiotic
Mykrox	Diuretic
Myleran	Antineoplastic
Mymethasone	Glucocorticoid
Myolin	Skeletal muscle relaxant
Mysoline	Barbiturate
Mytelase	Cholinesterase inhibitor
nabilone	Antiemetic
nabumetone	NSAID
nadolol	Beta blocker
Nadopen	Antibiotic
Nadostine	Antibiotic
Nafcil	Antibiotic
nafcillin	Antibiotic
naftifine	Antibiotic
Naftin	Antibiotic
Nalfon	NSAID
nalidixic acid	Antibiotic
Nallpen	Antibiotic
Napamide	Antidysrhythmic
Naprosyn	NSAID
naproxen	NSAID
Naqua	Diuretic
naratriptan	Antimigraine
Nardil	MAO inhibitor
Nasahist	Antihistamine
Nasalcrom	Mast cell stabilizer
Naturetin	Diuretic
Nauseatol	Antihistamine
Navane	Phenothiazine
Nebcin	Antibiotic

nedocromil	Mast cell stabilizer
nefazodone	SSRI antidepressant
NegGram	Antibiotic
nelfinavir	Antiviral agent
Nembutal	Barbiturate
neomycin	Antibiotic
Neoral	Immunosuppressant
neostigmine	Cholinesterase inhibitor
Neosynephrine	Decongestant
Neothylline	Methylxanthine bronchodilator
Neotrexin	Antineoplastic
Nephronex	Antibiotic
Neurotin	Anticonvulsant
nevirapine	Antiviral agent
Niazide	Diuretic
nicardipine	Calcium channel blocker
nifedipine	Calcium channel blocker
Nilandron	Antineoplastic
Nilstat	Antibiotic
nilutamide	Antineoplastic
nimodipine	Calcium channel blocker
Nimotop	Calcium channel blocker
Nisocor	Calcium channel blocker
nisoldipine	Calcium channel blocker
Nitro-Bid	Nitrate
Nitrocap	Nitrate
Nitrodisc	Nitrate
Nitro-Dur	Nitrate
Nitrofan	Antibiotic
nitrofurantoin	Antibiotic
Nitrogard	Nitrate
nitroglycerin	Nitrate
Nitroglyn	Nitrate
Nitrol	Nitrate

Nitrolingual	Nitrate
Nitrong	Nitrate
Nitrospan	Nitrate
Nitrostat	Nitrate
nizatidine	Antiulcer
Nizoral	Antibiotic
Nobesine	Anorexiant
Noctec	Anxiolytic
Noludar	Hypnotic
Nolvadex	Antineoplastic
norethindrone	Progesterone hormone
Norflex	Skeletal muscle relaxant
norfloxacin	Antibiotic
norgestrel	Estrogen hormone
Norlutin	Progesterone hormone
Normodyne	Beta blocker
Norometoprol	Beta blocker
Noroxin	Antibiotic
Norpace	Antidysrhythmic
Norplant	Progesterone hormone
Norpramin	Tricyclic antidepressant
nortriptyline	Tricyclic antidepressant
Norvasc	Calcium channel blocker
Norvir	Antiviral agent
Novamobarb	Barbiturate
Novamoxin	Antibiotic
Novo-Ampicillin	Antibiotic
novobiocin	Antibiotic
Novo-butamide	Oral hypoglycemic
Novochlorhydrate	Anxiolytic
Novochlorpromazine	Phenothiazine
Novoclopate	Benzodiazepine
Novocloxin	Antibiotic
Novocolchine	Uricosuric (antigout)

Novofibrate	Antihyperlipidemic
Novoflupam	Benzodiazepine
Novoflurazine	Phenothiazone
Novofuran	Antibiotic
Novohexidyl	Anticholinergic (antiparkinson)
Novolexin	Antibiotic
Novolin	Insulin preparation
Novopen	Antibiotic
Novopoxide	Benzodiazepine
Novopramine	Tricyclic antidepressant
Novopranol	Beta blocker
Novopurinol	Uricosuric (antigout)
Novoridazine	Phenothiazine
Novosalmol	Adrenergic bronchodilator
Novosorbide	Nitrate
Novospiroton	Diuretic
Novothalidone	Diuretic
Nozinan	Phenothiazine
Nyaderm	Antibiotic
nystatin	Antibiotic
Nysten	Antibiotic
octreotide	Antidiarrheal
Ocufen	NSAID
Ocuflox	Antibiotic
Ocupress	Beta blocker
ofloxacin	Antibiotic
Ogen	Estrogen hormone
Olanzapine	SSRI antipsychotic
olopatadine	Antihistamine
olsalazine	Antiulcer
omeprazole	Antiulcer
Omnicef	Antibiotic
Omnipen	Antibiotic

ondansetron	Antiemetic
Optimine	Antihistamine
Oradexon	Glucocorticoid
Orap	Antipsychotic
Orasone	Glucocorticoid
Orinase	Oral hypoglycemic
Orlaam	Narcotic analgesic
Ormazine	Phenothiazine
orphenadrine	Skeletal muscle relaxant
Orudis	NSAID
Oruvail	NSAID
Otrivin	Decongestant
Ovrette	Estrogen hormone
oxacillin	Antibiotic
oxazepam	Benzodiazepine
oxtriphylline	Methylxanthine bronchodilator
oxybutynin	Anticholinergic
oxycodone	Narcotic analgesic
Oxydess	CNS stimulant
oxytetracycline	Antibiotic
Pamelor	Tricyclic antidepressant
Pamine	Anticholinergic
Panasol	Glucocorticoid
pancrealipase	Digestant
Pancrease	Digestant
Panectyl	Antihistamine
Panmycin	Antibiotic
Panwarfin	Anticoagulant
papaverine	Vasodilator
Paracetaldehyde	Barbiturate
Paradione	Anticonvulsant
Paraflex	Skeletal muscle relaxant
Parafon Forte	Skeletal muscle relaxant
Paral	Barbiturate

paraldehyde	Barbiturate
paramethadione	Anticonvulsant
paramethasone	Glucocorticoid
paregoric	Antidiarrheal
Parlodel	Adrenergic bronchodilator
Parnate	MAO inhibitor
paromomycin	Antibiotic
paroxetine	SSRI antidepressant
Patanol	Antihistamine
Pathocil	Antibiotic
Pavabid	Vasodilator
Pavased	Vasodilator
Pavatyme	Vasodilator
Paxil	SSRI antidepressant
Paxipam	Benzodiazepine
Pelamine	Antihistamine
pemoline	CNS stimulant
Penbritin	Antibiotic
penbutolol	Beta blocker
penciclovir	Antiviral agent
Penetrex	Antibiotic
Penglobe	Antibiotic
penicillin	Antibiotic
pentaerythritol	Nitrate
Pentazine	Phenothiazine
pentazocine	Narcotic analgesic
pentobarbital	Barbiturate
pentoxifylline	Antiplatelet
Pentylan	Nitrate
Percocet	Narcotic analgesic
Percodan	Narcotic analgesic
pergolide	Antiparkinson
Pergonal	Infertility drug
Periactin	Antihistamine

Peridol	Antipsychotic
Perindopril	ACE inhibitor
Peritrate	Nitrate
Permax	Antiparkinson
perphenazine	Phenothiazine
Pertofrane	Tricyclic antidepressant
Pethadol	Narcotic analgesic
Pethidine	Narcotic analgesic
P.E.T.N.	Nitrate
Pfizerpen	Antibiotic
Phenazine	Phenothiazine
Phencen	Phenothiazine
phenelzine	MAO inhibitor
Phenergan	Phenothiazine
phenmetrazine	CNS stimulant
phenobarbital	Barbiturate
phenoxybenzamine	Alpha$_1$ blocker
phenylbutazone	NSAID
phenytoin	Anticonvulsant
pimozide	Antipsychotic
pindolol	Beta blocker
pipobroman	Antineoplastic
pirbuterol	Adrenergic bronchodilator
piroxicam	NSAID
Placidyl	Barbiturate
Plavix	Antiplatelet
Plendil	Calcium channel blocker
Poladex	Antihistamine
Polaramine	Antihistamine
Polargen	Antihistamine
Polycillin	Antibiotic
Polymox	Antibiotic
polymyxin	Antibiotic
polythiazide	Diuretic

Ponstan	NSAID
Ponstel	NSAID
pramipexole	Anticholinergic (antiparkinson)
Prandin	Oral hypoglycemic
Pravachol	Antihyperlipidemic
pravastatin	Antihyperlipidemic
prazocin	Alpha$_1$ blocker
Precose	Oral hypoglycemic
prednisolone	Glucocorticoid
prednisone	Glucocorticoid
Preludin	CNS stimulant
Premarin	Estrogen hormone
Prevacid	Antiulcer
Prevalyte	Antihyperlipidemic
Priftin	Antituberculosis agent
Prilosec	Antiulcer
primidone	Barbiturate
Principen	Antibiotic
Prinivil	ACE inhibitor
ProAmatine	Alpha$_1$ agonist
Proaqua	Diuretic
Probalan	Uricosuric (antigout)
Pro-Banthine	Antiulcer
probenecid	Uricosuric (antigout)
procainamide	Antidysrhythmic
Procan	Antidysrhythmic
Procanbid	Antidysrhythmic
procarbazine	Antineoplastic
Procardia	Calcium channel blocker
prochlorperazine	Phenothiazine
Procyclid	Anticholinergic (antiparkinson)
procyclidine	Anticholinergic (antiparkinson)

Progens	Estrogen hormone
progesterone	Progesterone hormone
Prograf	Immunosuppressant
Prolixin	Phenothiazine
Proloprim	Antibiotic
Promapar	Phenothiazine
Promaz	Phenothiazine
promazine	Phenothiazine
promethazine	Phenothiazine
Prometrium	Progesterone hormone
Pronestyl	Antidysrhythmic
propafanone	Antidysrhythmic
Propanthel	Antiulcer
propantheline	Antiulcer
Propion	Anorexiant
propoxyphene	Narcotic analgesic
propranolol	Beta blocker
Propulsid	Antireflux
Proren	Phenothiazine
Pro-Sof	Stool softener
Prosom	Benzodiazepine
Prostaphlin	Antibiotic
Prostigmin	Cholinesterase inhibitor
Protophylline	Methylxanthine bronchodilator
Protostat	Antibiotic
protriptyline	Tricyclic antidepressant
Proventil	Adrenergic bronchodilator
Provera	Progesterone hormone
Prozac	SSRI antidepressant
Prozine	Phenothiazine
pseudoephedrine	Decongestant
Pulmicort	Glucocorticoid
Pulmozyme	Mucolytic

Purinethol	Antineoplastic
Purinol	Uricosuric (antigout)
pyrazinamide	Antituberculosis agent
Pyribenzamine	Antihistamine
quazepam	Benzodiazepine
Questran	Antihyperlipidemic
quetiapine	SSRI antipsychotic
Quibron	Methylxanthine bronchodilator
Quiess	Antihistamine
quinacrine	Antibiotic
Quinaglute	Antidysrhythmic
quinapril	ACE inhibitor
Quinidex	Antidysrhythmic
quinidine	Antidysrhythmic
raloxifene	Estrogen hormone
ramipril	ACE inhibitor
rantidine	Antiulcer
Raxar	Antibiotic
Reactine	Antihistamine
Reglan	Cholinergic
Regulax	Stool softener
Regutol	Stool softener
Rela	Skeletal muscle relaxant
Relafen	NSAID
Remeron	Antidepressant
Renese	Diuretic
Renormax	ACE inhibitor
repaglinide	Oral hypoglycemic
Requip	Anticholinergic (antiparkinson)
Rescriptor	Antiviral agent
reserpine	Antihypertensive
Respbid	Methylxanthine bronchodilator

Restoril	Benzodiazepine
Retrovir	Antiviral agent
Rheumatrex	Antineoplastic
Rhinocort	Glucocorticoid
Rhodis	NSAID
ribavirin	Antiviral agent
rifabutin	Antituberculosis
Rifadin	Antituberculosis
rifampin	Antituberculosis
rifapentine	Antituberculosis
Rilutek	Anti-ALS
riluzole	Anti-ALS
Rimactane	Antituberculosis
rimantadine	Antiviral agent
Risperdal	Antipsychotic
risperidone	Antipsychotic
Ritalin	CNS stimulant
ritonavir	Antiviral agent
Rivotril	Benzodiazepine
rizatriptan	Antimigraine
Robaxin	Skeletal muscle relaxant
Robicillin	Antibiotic
Robidone	Narcotic analgesic
Robimycin	Antibiotic
Robinul	Antiulcer
Robitet	Antibiotic
Rofact	Antituberculosis
Rogaine	Vasodilator
ropinirole	Anticholinergic (antiparkinson)
Ro-sulfiram	Antialcohol
Roxicet	Narcotic analgesic
Roxicodone	Narcotic analgesic
RuVert-M	Antiemetic
Rynacrom	Mast cell stabilizer

Rythmodan	Antidysrhythmic
Rythmol	Antidysrhythmic
Salbutamol	Adrenergic bronchodilator
Salflex	NSAID
salmeterol	Adrenergic bronchodilator
salsalate	NSAID
Salsitab	NSAID
Saluron	Diuretic
Sandimmune	Immunosuppressant
Sansert	Antimigraine
saquinavir	Protease inhibitor
Sarisol	Barbiturate
scopolamine	Anticholinergic (antiparkinson)
secobarbital	Barbiturate
Seconal	Barbiturate
Sectral	Beta blocker
selegiline	MAO inhibitor
Semilente	Insulin preparation
senna	Laxative
Senokot	Laxative
Senolax	Laxative
Septra	Antibiotic
Serax	Benzodiazepine
Sereen	Benzodiazepine
Serentil	Phenothiazine
Serevent	Adrenergic bronchodilator
Seromycin	Antituberculosis agent
Seroquel	SSRI antipsychotic
Serpalan	Antihypertensive
sertraline	SSRI antidepressant
Serzone	SSRI antidepressant

sibutramine	Anorexiant
sildenafil	Vasodilator
simvastatin	Antihyperlipidemic
Sinemet	Anticholinergic (antiparkinson)
Sinequan	Tricyclic antidepressant
Singulair	Leukotriene blocker
Sinusol	Antihistamine
Slo-Bid	Methylxanthine bronchodilator
Slo-Phyllin	Methylxanthine bronchodilator
Solazine	Phenothiazone
Solfoton	Barbiturate
Solium	Benzodiazepine
Soma	Skeletal muscle relaxant
Somophyllin	Methylxanthine bronchodilator
Sonazine	Phenothiazine
Soprodol	Skeletal muscle relaxant
Sorbitrate	Nitrate
sotalol	Beta blocker
Spancap	CNS stimulant
sparfloxacin	Antibiotic
Sparine	Phenothiazine
Spectrobid	Antibiotic
spirapril	ACE inhibitor
spironolactone	Diuretic
Sporanox	Antibiotic
Staticin	Antibiotic
stavudine	Antiviral agent
Stelazine	Phenothiazone
Stilphostrol	Estrogen hormone
Stimate	Antidiuretic hormone
sucralfate	Antiulcer

Sudafed	Decongestant
Sular	Calcium channel blocker
sulfamethoxazole	Antibiotic
sulfinpyrazone	Uricosuric (antigout)
sulfisoxazole	Antibiotic
sulindac	NSAID
sumatriptan	Antimigraine
Sumox	Antibiotic
Sumycin	Antibiotic
Suprax	Antibiotic
Surmontil	Tricyclic antidepressant
Sustiva	Antiviral agent
Symmetrel	Anticholinergic (antiparkinson)
Synthroid	Thyroid hormone
Tace	Estrogen hormone
tacrine	Cholinesterase inhibitor
tacrolimus	Immunosuppressant
Talwin	Narcotic analgesic
Tambocor	Antidysrhythmic
Tamofen	Antineoplastic
tamoxifen	Antineoplastic
tamsulosin	Alpha$_1$ blocker
Tao	Antibiotic
Tapazole	Antithyroid agent
Taractan	Phenothiazine
Tarasan	Phenothiazine
Tasmar	Antiparkinson
Tebrazid	Antituberculosis agent
Tegopen	Antibiotic
Tegretol	Anticonvulsant
Temaril	Antihistamine
temazepam	Benzodiazepine
Tenex	Antihypertensive
Tenormin	Beta blocker

Ten-Tab	Anorexiant
Tenuate	Anorexiant
Tenuate Dospan	Anorexiant
Tepanil	Anorexiant
terazosin	$Alpha_1$ blocker
terbutaline	Adrenergic bronchodilator
Terfenadine	Antihistamine
Terfluzine	Phenothiazine
Terramycin	Antibiotic
Teslac	Antineoplastic
Tessalon	Antitussive
testolactone	Antineoplastic
tetracycline	Antibiotic
Tetracyn	Antibiotic
Tetralan	Antibiotic
Thalidomide	Immunosuppressant
Thalitone	Diuretic
Thalomid	Immunosuppressant
Theo-Dur	Methylxanthine bronchodilator
Theolair	Methylxanthine bronchodilator
theophylline	Methylxanthine bronchodilator
thiethylperazine	Antiemetic
thioridazine	Phenothiazine
thiothixene	Phenothiazine
Thorazine	Phenothiazine
Thor-Prom	Phenothiazine
Thylline	Methylxanthine bronchodilator
Thyrar	Thyroid hormone
thyroid	Thyroid hormone
Thyrolar	Thyroid hormone

tiagabine	Anticonvulsant
Tiamate	Calcium channel blocker
Tiazac	Calcium channel blocker
Ticar	Antibiotic
ticarcillin	Antibiotic
Ticlid	Antiplatelet
ticlopidine	Antiplatelet
Ticon	Antiemetic
Tigan	Antiemetic
Tilade	Mast cell stabilizer
timolol	Beta blocker
Tizanidine	Skeletal muscle relaxant
tobramycin	Antibiotic
Tobrex	Antibiotic
tocainamide	Antidysrhythmic
Tofranil	Tricyclic antidepressant
tolazamide	Oral hypoglycemic
tolbutamide	Oral hypoglycemic
tolcapone	Anticholinergic (antiparkinson)
Tolectin	NSAID
Tolinase	Oral hypoglycemic
tolmetin	NSAID
tolterodine	Anticholinergic
Tonocard	Antidysrhythmic
Topamax	Anticonvulsant
topiramate	Anticonvulsant
Toprol	Beta blocker
Toradol	NSAID
Torecan	Antiemetic
toremifene	Antineoplastic
Tornalate	Adrenergic bronchodilator
torsemide	Diuretic
Totacillin	Antibiotic

tramadol	Narcotic analgesic
Trandate	Beta blocker
trandolapril	ACE inhibitor
Tranxene	Benzodiazepine
tranylcypromine	MAO inhibitor
Travamine	Antihistamine
trazodone	Antidepressant
Trecator-SC	Antituberculosis
Trental	Antiplatelet
Triadapin	Tricyclic antidepressant
triamcinolone	Glucocorticoid
triamterene	Diuretic
triazolam	Benzodiazepine
Trichlorex	Diuretic
trichlormethiazide	Diuretic
Tricor	Antihyperlipidemic
Tridil	Nitrate
trifluoperazine	Phenothiazone
trifluridine	Antiviral agent
Trihexy	Anticholinergic (antiparkinson)
trihexyphenidyl	Anticholinergic (antiparkinson)
Trilafon	Phenothiazine
Trilisate	NSAID
trimeprazine	Antihistamine
trimethobenzamide	Antiemetic
trimethoprim	Antibiotic
trimetrexate	Antineoplastic
trimipramine	Tricyclic antidepressant
Trimox	Antibiotic
Trimoxazole	Antibiotic
Trimpex	Antibiotic
Trinalin	Antihistamine
tripelennamine	Antihistamine

triprolidine	Antihistamine
Triptil	Tricyclic antidepressant
Triptone	Anticholinergic (antiparkinson)
troleandomycin	Antibiotic
Tylenol	Analgesic
Ultracef	Antibiotic
Ultralente	Insulin preparation
Ultram	Narcotic analgesic
Ultrase	Digestant
Uni-Dur	Methylxanthine bronchodilator
Unipen	Antibiotic
Uniphyl	Methylxanthine bronchodilator
Univasc	ACE inhibitor
Urabeth	Cholinergic
Uracel	NSAID
uracil	Antineoplastic
Urecholine	Cholinergic
Urex	Antibiotic
Uridon	Diuretic
Urispas	Antidysrhythmic
Urofollitropin	Infertility drug
Urozide	Diuretic
Utimox	Antibiotic
valacyclovir	Antiviral agent
Valium	Benzodiazepine
valproic acid	Anticonvulsant
valsartan	Angiotensin II blocker
Valtrex	Antiviral agent
Vamate	Antihistamine
Vancenase	Glucocorticoid
Vanceril	Glucocorticoid

Vancocin	Antibiotic
Vancoled	Antibiotic
vancomycin	Antibiotic
Vantin	Antibiotic
Vascor	Calcium channel blocker
Vasodilan	Vasodilator
Vasoprine	Vasodilator
Vasotec	ACE inhibitor
V-Cillin	Antibiotic
Veetids	Antibiotic
Velosef	Antibiotic
Velosulin	Insulin preparation
venlafaxine	SSRI antidepressant
Ventolin	Adrenergic bronchodilator
verapamil	Calcium channel blocker
Vercyte	Antineoplastic
Verelan	Calcium channel blocker
Viagra	Vasodilator
Vibramycin	Antibiotic
Vicodin	Narcotic analgesic
Videx	Antiviral agent
Vimicon	Antihistamine
Viokase	Digestant
Viracept	Antiviral agent
Viramune	Antiviral agent
Virazole	Antiviral agent
Viroptic	Antiviral agent
Visken	Beta blocker
Vistacon	Antihistamine
Vistacrom	Mast cell stabilizer
Vistaril Oral	Antihistamine
Vivactil	Tricyclic antidepressant
Vivelle	Estrogen hormone

Vivol	Benzodiazepine
Vivox	Antibiotic
Volmax	Adrenergic bronchodilator
Voltaren	NSAID
Vontrol	Antivertigo
warfarin	Anticoagulant
Warfilone	Anticoagulant
Wellbutrin	Antidepressant
Wymox	Antibiotic
Wytensin	Antihypertensive
Xanax	Benzodiazepine
Xeloda	Antineoplastic
xylometazoline	Decongestant
zafirlukast	Leukotriene antagonist
Zagam	Antibiotic
zalcitabine	Antiviral agent
Zanaflex	Skeletal muscle relaxant
Zantac	Antiulcer
Zapex	Benzodiazepine
Zarontin	Anticonvulsant
Zaroxolyn	Diuretic
Zebeta	Beta blocker
Zerit	Antiviral agent
Zestril	ACE inhibitor
zidovudine	Antiviral agent
zileuton	Leukotriene antagonist
Zinacef	Antibiotic
Zithromax	Antibiotic
Zocor	Antihyperlipidemic
Zofran	Antiemetic
zolmitriptan	Antimigraine
Zoloft	SSRI antidepressant
zolpidem	Anxiolytic
Zomig	Antimigraine

Zonalon	Tricyclic antidepressant
Zovirax	Antiviral agent
Zyban	Antidepressant
Zydol	Narcotic analgesic
Zyflo	Leukotriene antagonist
Zyloprim	Uricosuric (antigout)
Zyprexa	SSRI antipsychotic
Zyrtec	Antihistamine

Note: Generic drug names appear in bold; classes of drugs in all uppercase letters. Italicized page numbers denote a definition.

Z